DEDICATION

This book is dedicated to Wendie Joe Sperber,
founder of weSPARK, a Cancer Support Center and
its staff members and volunteers.

http://www.wespark.org

"It is not how many years we live, but rather what we do with them."
- Evangeline Cory Booth

Making the Breast of It

Overcoming Fear of Intimacy
After Mastectomy

Lea Yekutiel

MAKING THE BREAST OF IT

Overcoming Fear of Intimacy After Mastectomy

Published by:
Who Am I Press
4444 Hazeltine Ave. #229
Sherman Oaks, CA 91423 USA

lea@ilovemybreastcancer.com
http://www.ilovemybreastcancer.com

First printing 2007

Copyright © 2007 by Lea Yekutiel
Printed in the United States of America

Library of Congress Cataloging-in-Publication Data
Yekutiel, Lea.

2007924991

Making the Breast of It: Overcoming Fear
of Intimacy After Mastectomy / Lea Yekutiel

ISBN 0-9774174-0-9

ENDORSEMENT

"Let her help you and the world end breast cancer."

Mark Victor Hansen - co-author of the series "Chicken Soup for the Soul"

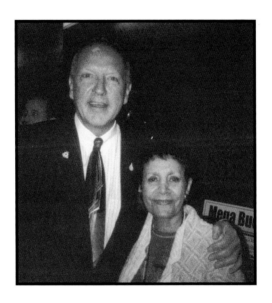

Mark Victor Hansen and Lea Yekutiel
Los Angeles, CA
March 2007

TABLE OF CONTENTS

Acknowledgments   XI
Warning-Disclaimer   XII
Foreword   XIII
My Inspiration   XV

Chapter 1: Silent Messenger   17
Finally, I Listen and Take Action   19
"M" for Malignant   22
Shaking with Fear   23
The Next Surgery   25

**Chapter 2: From Lumpectomy to
Mastectomy**   27
More Questions, Decisions and Confusion   28
It All Seemed Barbaric   29
Weighing My Options   30
Still Alone   32
Judgment Day   34
Highs and Lows—On My Chest   36
My Nightmare Continued   37
A Vicious Cycle   40
Let Go and Let God   41

Chapter 3: Taking Charge   43
My Angel, Diane   44
Threads Woven Into the Fabric of Life   47

Chapter 4: No Longer Feeling Alone   49
Finding Sanctuary   50

Chapter 5: Self-Acceptance 53
Baring My Soul's Purpose 55
My Mission Revealed on Stage 57
How the Universe Delivers 61
Law of Attraction 62
The Source of Fear of Intimacy 63
Negative Reactions from Men 67
Stories of Unconditional Love for Women After
Mastectomy 68
My Own Experiences 70

Chapter 6: Knowledge Is Power 77
How Our Conscious Mind Operates 81
How Our Subconscious Mind Works 83
The Conflict 85
Change Your Attitude, Change Your Life 86
Our Body Is Our Castle 88
A Gem Needs Polishing to Shine 89
Meditation and Happiness 91
Befriend Your Body 93
Benefits of Meditation 93
The Healing Power of Solitude 93
You Are Priceless 95

Chapter 7: The Will to Survive 97
Balance and Harmony 97
Blessing in Disguise 99
Never Failing Faith and Hope 101
The Comeback Kid 103

Chapter 8: My Two Mothers 107
My Biological Mother 107

A New Motherland   109
Home Without a Home   110
My Spiritual Mother   113
Virginia, the Healer   114
Compassion Exercise   116
An Exercise of Forgiveness   117
Gratitude Exercise   119
Virginia Leaves the Earth   120

**Chapter 9: Spiritual Beings Having a Human
Experience**   123
Nurturing Your Body   123
Nurturing Exercise   124
Meditation Exercise
The Power of Solitude   125
Solitude Exercise   125
Ancient Chinese Healing Acupuncture   126
Body, Mind, Spirit Activities   127

Afterword   133

Appendix A   135
Compassion Exercise   135
Forgiveness Exercise   136
Simple Concentration Exercises   137
Gratitude Exercise   137
Nurturing Exercise   137
Meditation Exercise   138
Body, Mind, Spirit Activities   140
Ten Ways to Honor Your Uniqueness   145
Living in the Moment   149
Attention and Focus   152

Appendix B   **155**
weSPARK Mission   **155**
weSPARK Founder   **155**

ACKNOWLEDGMENTS

I would like to thank the following very special people: Tara Shore the instructor from my creative writing group at weSPARK. Without your input and encouragement this book would not have come to existence. Tara, you helped me to get on the right track. I'd like also to thank all the participants in our creative writing group. I have learned a great deal from your talents. Also, to my dearest friends Nancy Allen and Patricia Stewart at weSpark I wish to express deep gratitude.

I'd like to thank my brother, Mordechai Yekutiel, who supported me in many different ways to bring this book into print.

I would like to express my thanks to my aunt, Tamar Yekutiel, who always managed to keep the family together, and for her devotion to my grandfather. I admire you for your dedication.

"Thank you" to my sister Sara Green who called from England a few times a month to check up on me throughout the year of all my surgeries.

Another big "thank you" to my girlfriend, Rivka Horowitz, who faithfully came to visit me every day after work for three months. She kept calling me every evening for over a year to make sure I was ok.

I'd like to thank Sam Horn, the author of many books and a guru of creating book titles. She is responsible for helping me to choose the title of this book.

Another word of appreciation to Tammy Takahashi and especially to Veronica Sauter, Ph.D. for helping me with editing this book.

And last but not least to my book cover designer, Ramesh Choudhary, who is also responsible for the layout of the book and who accommodated my many requests. Thank you!

WARNING—DISCLAIMER

This book is a personal account of my journey and experiences with cancer and with the doctors who treated me. Your experience may be totally different.

The purpose of this book is to empower, encourage and inspire the reader to never give up hope.

It is not the purpose of this book to give the reader any medical advice or claim that Eastern Medicine is better or superior than Western Medicine.

The narrative and the information in this book are in the nature of guidance and geared more toward personal development and spiritual growth. It is not a substitute for seeking professional medical help.

Every effort has been made to use fictitious names for both the doctors who treated me and the institutions where care was administered.

The author shall have neither liability nor responsibility to any person or entity with respect to any loss or damage caused, or alleged to have been caused, directly or indirectly, by the information contained in this book.

If you do not wish to be bound by the above, you may return this book to the publisher for full refund.

FOREWORD

Above all, life is an emotional experience. It is what some call 'the human experience.' This condition is both our strength and our weakness, and all of our human behavior hinges on the challenge of exploring certain emotions. In many ways, emotions are the fuel which powers our lives. It is also emotions that bind us together, for on this level we all experience the same set of emotions. Different events may provoke or stimulate different emotions in each of us. In this, we differ from each other, yet we all react out of the same set of human emotions.

Though many of us would like to think that love is our strongest emotion, I doubt this to be true. I suspect that fear is our strongest emotion. We are all afraid of many things and of different things for different reasons. Some of our fears are biological, others are psychological. Some fears are real and many are imagined. One fear I believe we all share is the fear of being alone. We are all capable of facing and handling many of life's traumas, but the thought of doing it alone is often overwhelming. As part of my work, I do a lot of flying, and I often think about the possibility of a crash. As I contemplate these thoughts, I always realize that the worst thing would be if there were not a person seated next to me whose hand I could reflexively touch as we were going down.

Illness is always accompanied by fear: the fear of pain and suffering, the fear of deformity, the fear of being a burden to others and the fear of death itself are all common. Each and every step on the journey of healing from an illness appears far more distressing and overwhelming when we have to face it alone. It is at times such as these that human want and human need are felt most deeply. It is at such times that even the strongest among us welcome a human touch, a kind word, a shoulder to cry on, help with practical chores, and someone to make us feel we are not alone. Even a stranger is welcomed.

Ms. Lea Yekutiel's voice speaks clearly to this basic human need as she describes her journey through her experience with breast cancer. Though this journey is her own, it belongs to all of us. It reminds all of us just how vulnerable we are. A diagnosis of breast cancer adds a particular fear for women who are treated with mastectomy; namely, the fear of loss of sexual attractiveness. This is not a minor issue, nor is it an issue restricted to younger women, as some would like to believe. It is not an issue of vanity. It is universal and it is deep. It is rarely discussed. Its roots are grounded in emotional bedrock—in loneliness—the fear of being alone.

As the story of Ms. Yekutiel unfolds, you discover that she finds the answer to her *question, "God. Cancer. How is it possible that this is happening to me?"* It is a common answer, and it represents self-acceptance and ultimately self-growth. The answer is simple. It is being of service to others. It is in this role that we are most satisfied. It is in this way that we feel our best and that we are our best. It is through service that we are connected to others, and in so doing we feel less alone.

Silvana Martino, D.O.
Director, Breast Cancer Program
The Angeles Clinic and Research Institute

MY INSPIRATION

This is not just another cancer story. If my sole intention were to tell another story about breast cancer, I would have stopped right there. Instead, I want to tell my story with a fresh slant.

I would like to tell my story of overcoming the fear of intimacy after mastectomy through my spiritual training. It is a story of how I became a stronger human being because of my experience, and how it can help women enjoy an intimate life with the opposite sex after breast cancer or mastectomy. It is a story of inspiration, hope, empowerment, encouragement, and never ever giving up—a story of how to honor yourself and grow spiritually.

Most of all, it's a story of how you, too, can accept yourself completely and enjoy feeling like a whole woman—with one breast or with none.

In Africa, there is a tribe in which expectant mothers create a song-of-the-soul for their unborn children. Villagers sing this song to the baby at birth and at every important moment of his life--from his first step to his wedding day. The song is also sung when that person steps out of the integrity of his true self. Rather than be punished, the individual is brought back into harmony through the music of his soul. You, too, have a soul song that belongs only to you. Listen for it. Re-discover the harmony of your own life.

- Mary Manin Morrissey

CHAPTER 1

Silent Messenger

"Trusting your intuition means tuning in as deeply as you can to the energy you feel, following that energy moment to moment, trusting that it will lead you where you want to go and bring you everything you desire."
— Shakti Gawain

As I sat in a lounge chair outside a house on the top of a mountain overlooking the Pacific Ocean, breezes whispered on my skin. I was surrounded by a riot of flowers: deep red roses, yellow lilies, pink cherry blossoms, orange birds of paradise, sunflowers, carnations, tulips, daisies, daffodils, and gardenias. The scent of a nearby avocado orchard drifted toward my nose.

On this sunny summer afternoon, I was on a Spiritual Quest at a retreat center in the small town of Montecito near Santa Barbara, California.

Although I may have looked lazy sitting in my lounge chair, I was actively meditating, practicing spiritual exercises to shed excess baggage and eliminate beliefs that didn't serve me anymore. I wanted to reach a state of clarity.

Normally, when I did spiritual exercises, I enjoyed a state of euphoria, my mind clear, my spirit light; nothing bothered me. Yet, as I soaked in this natural beauty, usually so restorative, I felt a dark cloud covering me. A negative and oppressive vibration was clinging to my body, mostly on my left side. I looked around but couldn't see anything. I felt strange.

In an attempt to rid myself of this unsettling feeling, I gestured to push this vibration away. "Get away from me! Get away," I said out loud for no one but the flowers to hear.

The dark cloud persistently enveloped me. *How could I attract this negative vibration on such a beautiful day in these* magnificent *surroundings?* It was perplexing.

I attempted to ignore the weird feeling and continued my spiritual exercises, but I couldn't concentrate. Like a tongue probing a painful tooth, my mind kept wandering back to the vibration.

A half-hour later, I was still unable to explain this strange experience felt tingling on the upper part of my left breast. *Was my Higher Self trying to tell me something? If so, what?*

Next, I tried "discreation," a way to uncreate unwanted or undesirable feelings that don't serve me anymore. The discreation process involves three steps.

1. I concentrate on a particular image of anger or sadness from my past that still disturbs me. I experience deep inside how that image feels from every angle. I stay with that image until I reach its edges.
2. I let the image dissolve.
3. I disassociate or disconnect from that image. After taking these three steps, the image just disappears.

But this time, the discreation process I had always relied on didn't work. I still couldn't concentrate.

Finally I Listen and Take Action

A month after this experience at the retreat center, I felt a murmuring sensation going through my upper left breast. *How odd.* I touched the area and felt a bit of hardness. I touched my right breast on the same spot and I felt the same kind of hardness just like the left side. That negative vibration I'd felt on the mountaintop had continued to follow me all this time. At that point, I picked up the phone to schedule an appointment to see a doctor. Impulsively, I changed my mind and hung up.

Another month passed and once again I felt something happening in my left breast, this time with slight pain. I'd heard that pain is not one of the symptoms of cancer. I also didn't feel a lump like most cancer patients do, so I let it go. But despite this rationalization, the dark cloud and unsettling vibrations were still consuming me.

Finally, I set up an appointment for a mammogram. A week after this mammogram, I got a call from the mammogram department at the hospital saying that the radiologist wanted me to schedule another mammogram. He had spotted something abnormal in my left breast and wanted to make sure that his observation was correct. After this mammogram the radiologist told me on the spot that he was certain I had an abnormality in my left breast.

My next appointment was to see a breast surgeon, Dr. Johnson. To my surprise, this doctor was tall and handsome—simply gorgeous. In his late thirties or early forties, his looks matched every woman's dream (including mine) of male perfection. He examined me and concluded that I needed to have a biopsy to determine the cause of the abnormality detected on the two mammograms.

I panicked. Biopsy? I didn't even know what that meant. I was in my mid-fifties. I'd never been hospitalized or gone through any kind of surgery. I felt scared and very isolated, especially because I was all alone without close friends or family members nearby. There was nobody I could talk with or lean on for support. It was up to the doctors and me alone—or so it seemed.

I had so much to learn. I didn't know that having a biopsy meant I had to have surgery and go under anesthesia. But before he could do a biopsy, the breast surgeon had to know exactly where the abnormality was, so I had to go through a humiliating and painful examination that lasted for hours.

First, a mammography technician gave me a hospital gown that was open in the front. She led me to a room with all kinds of machines. *What a cold, mechanical environment it was,* I thought. Then she attempted to inject dye through a vein in my breast. This attempt took a while since she could not find a vein in which to inject the dye. This was very painful because it was done without sedation. I was told the mammogram was needed so the surgeon would know which breast tissue he'd have to take for a biopsy. Then the technician pressed my breast between two glass plates to allow this machine to take an X-ray from every angle. Imagine a pancake maker into which you pour batter and press the top part down to image it. In this case, it was my breast in the pancake maker, squashed between two cold metallic plates. I felt like my breast was a "piece of meat," a separate part of my body.

After that, I had to prepare for the biopsy itself. The whole environment in the preparation room for the surgery frightened me. The nurse started with injections and connected my arm to an intravenous drip solution meant to help me relax. It actually made me numb so the doctors could mark my breast.

Next, they wheeled me into an operating room. The last thing I heard one of the nurses say was: "It's margarita time." I think I was still conscious because I replied in disbelief, "I am going to surgery and you are talking about a margarita?" Then she placed a mask on my nose, which put me out under general anesthesia. (Many months later, I learned that when the nurse said "margarita," she meant the anesthesia she was giving me. I've sure learned a lot since then.)

In the recovery room, I recall hearing muffled voices around me. I was in excruciating pain and crying for help, but no one came to my rescue. It seemed like hours passed. Finally, I felt someone slapping my cheeks. *I guess that's how they wake up their patients.* Then someone else gave me a painkiller.

After a while, another person came to pick me up from the hospital and dropped me at home—I don't even know who that was. But I do know the nurses sent me home with tubes coming out of my breast to drain blood and other fluids from the oozing incision. I felt like a monster, a creature from another world. I didn't even want to imagine how I looked!

During the week following my biopsy, I stayed fairly calm and tapped into my naturally positive nature. By this time, I'd heard stories about many biopsy results being negative and lumps benign. I prayed that my results would be negative as well.

"M" for Malignant

A week after the biopsy, I received a call from Dr. Johnson. Boy, did I have a crush on him, fantasizing about having an affair with him as if an affair with a doctor would remedy the abnormality in my breast.

When I first heard his voice, I wanted him to tell me all my worries were in vain that I could throw them out the window. Unfortunately, I could tell by his serious tone that Dr. Johnson had something different in mind. Any crazy fantasy about having an affair with him vanished.

He informed me that the biopsy showed the abnormality was, in fact, malignant and he wanted to see me immediately. *Is that what the spiritual warning on that mountaintop was about? Had that been an intuition, a hunch, an inner knowing of what was to come?* I was in disbelief, yet deep down I knew that the weird feelings I experienced on that mountain had been an omen.

Dr. Johnson asked me to bring somebody with me to the appointment. That request alarmed me. If he wanted me to bring another person with me, it must mean he thought I couldn't handle the news alone and would need emotional support.

Shocked, I hung up the phone as my mind raced in denial and confusion. *Cancer. God, what was I thinking? How could I have brought this on myself! It must be a mistake! Impossible! I couldn't be a cancer candidate. Nobody in my family has had cancer. I'm 5' 3" with a good weight of 115 pounds. I eat healthy foods. I'm physically, spiritually, and mentally active. I don't even feel sick.*

The hardest part was that I was alone—nobody around to give me advice or share the fears and anxieties I was experiencing. Because I didn't have anyone close who was available to go with me to the doctor's appointment, I called Simone, the manager of the building where I lived. I asked if she would go with me. She agreed.

At my next appointment, Dr. Johnson told me that I would have to go through another surgery—a lumpectomy to remove the part of my breast that was infiltrated with the cancer cells. *What? Another surgery within ten days of the biopsy?* Again I thought that was impossible. *How could I handle this?*

I felt still more depressed, even though I was taking antidepressants already. I couldn't sleep. I cried constantly. The doctors and the nurses didn't know what to do with me.

I worried continually. *How could I live with Dr. Johnson removing part of my breast?* I was happy with the size of my breasts. I didn't even know what size I was when they asked me because I hadn't worn a bra in the last thirty years. (I learned I was a size C.) I'd never liked having anything pressed against my body and happily got away without wearing one.

Shaking with Fear

Eight days after the biopsy and two days before the lumpectomy, my whole body started shaking with fear. I'd never before experienced any kind of fear like that. My body clearly didn't want to go through another surgery so soon.

So I called Virginia, my spiritual master who lived an hour's drive away from me. With tears rolling down my cheeks, I told her about my diagnosis. She insisted I come up to Montecito to see her immediately for a healing session. I told her my legs were shaking so terribly, I knew I couldn't drive, so she encouraged me to find someone to drive me. I managed to ask a girlfriend and off we went. She dropped me off at Virginia's house with a promise to come back within an hour or two.

My intuition told me that my shaking body was a manifestation of a debilitating fear that had been dominating my life. But I didn't know what to do about it. An exercise I did with Virginia helped me to find the source of that fear. She simply asked me, "What are you afraid of?" I searched in my heart for an answer to her question and realized that I was afraid of losing my independence. I lived alone with no family or close friends for support. Having grown up to be self-sufficient, I was afraid to become dependent on someone despite the illness I was facing.

Here's what I experienced following Virginia's question.

First, I "felt the feeling" of having to be dependent on someone else. I tuned in to acutely sense how it felt.

Next, I experienced and "felt the feeling" of not having to be dependent on someone else, and fully experienced how that felt.

Lastly, I experienced and felt both scenarios simultaneously. I began to struggle. A fight was going on in my mind between the two.

I did this exercise for about 15 minutes until I accepted the fact that it was okay to depend on others sometimes. As soon as I accepted that, my shaking stopped. By the time my girlfriend picked me up, she could tell I was as calm as a lamb. She could hardly believe her eyes. My body no longer trembled and my mind was filled with serenity and peacefulness.

The Next Surgery

The night before the lumpectomy, feelings of restlessness replaced the calm. I kept visualizing part of my left breast being cut off and getting smaller. *How would I be able to deal with that?* I couldn't think rationally. In fact, I was *afraid* to think; I'd rather be numb and not have to feel anything. I preferred that feeling to the pain I'd been experiencing.

The morning of the surgery, my elderly friend Bob picked me up to drive me to the hospital. On the way there, we talked about everything except the surgery. When we arrived, surprisingly I was calm and light as if the weight of all my worries had magically lifted from my shoulders. What a relief it was. I even asked the person who signed me in for surgery if he knew a good joke. I needed laughter in my life in order to relieve the pain, recognizing that laughter helps heal people.

During surgery, Dr. Johnson removed a large section of my left breast, making the difference in size between my two breasts seem tremendous. It was obvious to me that *I wouldn't be comfortable going braless anymore*.

Afterward, my positive attitude vanished. It couldn't help me face this whole ordeal. I was living in a state of haze and confusion. I would look at my new body, but couldn't recognize it as being mine—it had to be someone else's. Most of all, I felt lost and sad that I had so little control over what was going on in my life. And for the second time, I left the hospital with tubes coming out of my breast.

CHAPTER 2

From Lumpectomy to Mastectomy

"You gain strength, courage, and confidence by every experience in which you really stop to look fear in the face. You must do the thing which you think you cannot do."
— Eleanor Roosevelt

Ten days after the lumpectomy, I received another call from Dr. Johnson informing me that "the margins weren't clear." Would I again bring somebody with me to my next appointment?

What did it mean that the margins were not clear? I hated feeling ignorant about my medical issues and I didn't think I could handle any more bad news. In addition to living in uncertainty, confusion, and depression, I had to learn so many new medical terms. Yet I felt too overwhelmed and fatigued to investigate all my concerns. Nothing made sense. And again, I had to find someone to go with me to the next appointment. *Whom can I ask to go with me this time?*

It was torture to have to ask another elderly neighbor to accompany me to my appointment because it confirmed my social isolation and, in truth, my deep sense of loneliness. Thankfully, my elderly neighbor Abigail agreed to go with me.

We sat in Dr. Johnson's office. I was crying while he explained that I needed a mastectomy. *Mastectomy? What was that besides another new word that I had to add to my medical vocabulary?* Again I was in shock,

27

everything blurred in my mind. He continued with his explanation about the margins not being clear and not knowing exactly which part of my breast had more cancer cells. I still didn't understand.

It finally registered that the doctor wanted to remove my whole breast as soon as possible. I felt like it was just a bad dream. *If I can just wake up from this dream, everything will be fine.* I wanted to flee from the doctor's office, believing my problems would disappear, too. No wonder they told me to bring somebody with me to the appointment!

In all this confusion, I managed to ask, "Dr. Johnson, how much time do I have?"

"Three months," he answered.

That's all the time I have left to live on this earth?

Within seconds, my whole life rolled before my eyes in slow motion like a bad dream. *I have so many things I still want to do in this lifetime! I'm not ready to die!*

At that moment, the doctor saw my mounting panic and, with a knowing smile, clarified his words by saying, "You have three months to decide about the mastectomy." He also explained to me that there were some options available to me in the form of plastic surgery and implants.

More Questions, Decisions, and Confusion

Dr. Johnson told me that, if I wanted, he'd set up an appointment for me to see a plastic surgeon. The word "plastic surgeon" made a shiver run up and down my spine. *What was he really saying? He'd remove my breast—my flesh and blood, my pride as a woman— and insert a piece of plastic in its place? Would I ever date or enjoy intimacy with a lover again?* The doctor responded to my thoughts by saying, "Don't worry. This kind of surgery is a "piece of cake." It is done every day. *Easy for him to say! It's my body, not his.*

During this next period of getting examined by doctors and filling out questionnaires, I learned that one cause of breast cancer might be the hormone therapy I was on to help me with menopause. I was ordered to stop this therapy immediately. I also learned that the hormone therapy often comes with another side effect: depression. Yes, I'd been very depressed many months before my breast cancer diagnosis.

This news came as another shock to my system. Ten years before, my previous physician had put me on hormone therapy. *Now it's causing me to lose one of my breasts and suffer severe depression.*

To lift me out of my depression, I had been given antidepressant medication. *Living with depression meant I didn't have control over my emotions. I could burst into tears at any moment. Not* only did I lose control over my body, but over my feelings, too.

It All Seemed Barbaric

For a new century that lauded the most advanced medical care, my experience seemed so barbaric. Already in this journey, all that Western medical practice had caused me was more harm than good. They must have forgotten the Hippocratic oath, "First, do no harm."

The bewildering cycle was continuing. I was constantly crying, running from one doctor to the next, feeling hopeless, and seeking additional opinions, although in truth I didn't really know what I was looking for. Maybe I was praying that one doctor would tell me I'd been misdiagnosed and didn't have cancer after all.

I was living in such denial that when I received Dr. Johnson's referral to a plastic surgeon I tossed it into the trash. *Out of sight, out of mind,* I thought. But I realized I wasn't kidding anyone but myself! A week later, with shaking hands and a heavy heart, I dug through the trash, found the phone number, and set up an appointment with the plastic surgeon.

I couldn't imagine my body with only one breast. Unlike many women who never find satisfaction with their bodies, I loved my figure, my naturally olive skin, and my physical appearance. I used to wear flashy bikini swimsuits. I could easily pass as a teenager and attract the attention of men. Even in my early fifties, my figure always boosted my ego as a woman, and I didn't want that to change.

Maybe my ego was what finally convinced me to see the plastic surgeon. Yet, as soon as I went to his office and saw the "Plastic Surgeon" sign on the office door, I wanted to flee. I must have walked back and forth along that corridor for at least 15 minutes before I felt brave enough to walk in.

Weighing My Options

I was surprised how nonchalant the plastic surgeon, Dr. Pearson, came across. For him, I was just another patient, another case. For me, my breast was the most important part of my female anatomy.

Dr. Pearson started by methodically showing me slides of women who had mastectomies and the results of his work. He offered two options: One was an implant, which called for implanting a tissue expander under the skin and then injecting saline into it every two weeks; the second was a tram plant, a procedure that uses the patient's own tissues to rebuild a shapely breast. This procedure is much more complicated because of taking internal abdominal tissue from the woman's body to form a breast. The nine-hour surgery weakens the abdominal muscles.

I couldn't concentrate at all and cried through the entire appointment. Fortunately, I'd brought a tape recorder with me so I could replay the doctor's explanations about my options once I was thinking clearly. I knew it would help me get answers to the endless questions I would have following the appointment.

Later, I realized that doctors don't give their patients the whole picture about the many complications that might arise. They act like God, confidently showing that they "know it all." At least that's how this doctor acted.

After visiting with the plastic surgeon, I felt more confused than ever. Still living in denial, I was unable to replay the tape because I couldn't grasp or accept the seriousness of my situation. Added to denial was numbness because of all the antidepressant medication I was taking.

A few weeks passed and I had done nothing to decide about the plastic surgery. So I talked with a cancer nurse, Dina, about my dilemma. She put me in touch with a cancer patient who had tram plant surgery. I met with her and learned that she was happy with the results of her surgery. This gave me encouragement. However, after a second appointment with Dr. Pearson, I decided to have the implant procedure.

I chose to have the implant immediately following my mastectomy for two reasons. The main reason was to avoid waiting at least three months to let my body heal before having the implant surgery. I knew I couldn't face looking at myself in the mirror with only one breast for three whole months. The second reason was to avoid going under anesthesia so many times. Little did I know what was yet to happen.

Still Alone

Before mastectomy surgery, the hospital required me to sign a form called a "directive" that assigns a person to make decisions in case of complications during the surgery. As I mentioned, I was alone and had no one close I could ask to sign such a paper and assume the responsibility it implied.

Reluctantly, I mustered my courage and asked an elderly man named David who I knew from a club where we were both members. To my surprise, he agreed. He came over and signed the papers in the presence of the managers of the building. Then the day before my surgery, I called to tell him when we had to be at the hospital. He said he had to work and couldn't take me after all.

What was I going to do? Who could I ask at the last minute to drive me to the hospital? With my whole world caving in on me, everything seemed hopeless and cruel.

I felt angry because David never called after my surgery to find out how I was doing. Even when I saw him at the club, he never apologized or mentioned a word about his behavior. *What a cold world—people having no respect for one another and their words meaning nothing.* Once again, I had to rely on my spiritual tools and forgive this man who chose to work for a buck instead of keeping his word to me. It wasn't easy, but I knew that holding any grudges against him would just hurt me in the end.

Eventually I called Pearl, a woman I knew from group therapy, and asked her if she'd be willing to take me to the hospital for my surgery. A petite woman, Pearl was a gem just like her name implied. She graciously said "Yes." Because we had to be at the hospital early in the morning and she lived closer to the hospital than I did, she offered to pick me up the evening before and have me stay at her house overnight. She fed me and tucked me into bed like a young child. In the morning, she drove me to the hospital and made a point of being there when I awoke from the surgery.

I spent one night at the hospital and was released the next day. Pearl picked me up and insisted that I spend another night at her house so she could keep an eye on me. Again, she fed me and took care of me until she was sure that I could take care of myself. Thank goodness for Pearl. She restored my faith in people. After this, I always remember the saying, "When one door closes, another one opens."

Up to this point, I had not spoken about my situation to any members of my family. They lived far away in Israel, so I figured there was no reason for them to worry since they couldn't help me anyway. However, once I decided to go through with the mastectomy, I called one of my sisters to let her know about my situation. My mother, who was still alive at that time, was never told what I was going through. My sisters never said anything to her about me because she was not well. Knowing about my situation wouldn't help either of us.

I had the mastectomy and the implant at the same time, which meant Dr. Johnson performed the mastectomy and Dr. Pearson did the implant. The last memory I have of Dr. Johnson was in the operating room scrubbing his hands in preparation for removing my left breast.

Judgment Day

My anxiety didn't end with my mastectomy and implant. I was living in two different worlds, constantly switching from my own positive "all will be well" attitude to a worried state. Thankfully, the crying spells had stopped, giving me more control over my life.

My other world was the rising anxiety and fear imposed on me every time I had a doctor's appointment. It seemed like I was on a trial as a defendant with my doctors being the judges and members of the jury. My life depended on what happened on a particular day in the courtroom. *Would the testimonies be for me or against me? What will happen next?*

Here's an example of 'Judgment Day' in my mind. I called the first day I had to deal with the oncologist face to face 'Judgment Day' knowing the judge-appointed oncologist will read the verdict. After my mastectomy and implant, I had an appointment to see an oncologist—another new word I had to add to my vocabulary. Up to that point, I didn't know what role an oncologist played in the whole cancer treatment process. Nevertheless, intuitively I knew this doctor's part was important.

Feeling shaky, I sat in the crowded reception room with about fifteen other people waiting for the nurse to call our names. With every person the nurse called forward, I became more and more anxious. Most of them had come for chemotherapy treatments. It could be me the next time—all depending on the oncologist's verdict.

Finally, the nurse announced my name. I stood up and she led me to the doctor's office for my examination. The doctor pleasantly asked questions, examined me thoroughly, and then pronounced his verdict. Yes, for the first time during my ordeal, this doctor delivered a favorable ruling for me. He told me: "If you had the ability to choose the type of cancer to deal with, you chose the best one." *Perhaps he agrees with my beliefs that whatever we experience in life is our own creation and our own choosing,* I thought.

He told me that after the mastectomy, all the cancer cells were gone, that I had clear margins and a clean bill of health and didn't need to see an oncologist anymore. I would not have to go through chemotherapy or radiation. However, to make sure, the oncologist said I could take pills called Tamoxifen. "No," I replied immediately. "I don't want to put any more toxins into my body." *Toxic drugs from the hormone therapy brought me to this world of surgeries and doctors in the first place. How could I forget that?* The doctor agreed with me and said, "If I were you, I wouldn't take them either."

This oncologist was the only doctor I encountered who didn't try to prescribe any more pills for me to take. I was happy that I didn't have to go through chemotherapy or radiation or take more medication. *Wow, what a relief! What a glorious day!*

However, 'Judgment Day' hadn't completely passed me by.

Highs and Lows—On My Chest

I went to see the plastic surgeon every few weeks for follow-up. On one of these visits, Dr. Pearson wasn't there but I got bad news from the doctor who had stepped in. He told me that my implant had been positioned too high on my chest. *What? My doctor did not know where the implant should be placed on my chest?* I was very angry. This meant going through yet another surgery.

By now, I had concluded that I was dealing with butchers instead of professional doctors. My frustration and disappointments were mounting, especially because it was summertime when I was normally physically active. I couldn't do any exercises including swimming, which I loved. So in the afternoons, I'd sit by the pool in the shade and watch the sun shimmering on the water, constantly beckoning me to get in.

It wasn't enough that I wasn't allowed to swim, but I couldn't even move my arm as a result of removing some lymph nodes. I wasn't alone in my misery. As company I had my elderly neighbors who kept talking about their illnesses and their life histories. I actually felt older than them. Not being able to do anything physical reinforced this feeling.

This perpetual negative attitude frightened me. I'd always taken pride in my positive outlook. But these days, my head and feelings in my heart made me just like these older women who constantly complained about their lives. Even more frightening was wondering whether I'd survive long enough to reach their age. This marked a sad time during my recovery. What kept me going was my resolve to follow Virginia's teachings.

Also, I did anything I could to keep my attention off my body and the pain I was experiencing physically and emotionally. I joined Toastmasters International, an organization that would improve my public speaking. I started taking an art class to learn painting on ceramics. I painted vases that I gave to people as gifts or kept for myself. I took a sculpture class to learn sculpting figures in clay. I often went to the movies, which helped me escape for a while. But then I'd come home to an empty apartment and watch TV. I craved having a close relationship, being with someone who really cared about me and loved me, a warm human touch instead of those cold hospital rooms and doctors.

My wishes came true when one of my girlfriends, Rivka Horowitz (Ricki is her nick name), contacted me as soon as she found out about my situation. She started coming to my house almost every day after work to keep me company. She helped me wash my hair because I wasn't supposed to take showers. I remember telling her that she will be the only one who sees me in this situation. And for more than a year, she called me every night to check up on me. Thank goodness for Ricki!

My Nightmare Continued

About this time, I learned I would have to go through another surgery and hoped and prayed that this time, the doctor would insert the implant in the correct position on my chest.

Each surgery required a period of three months for my body to heal from the trauma of the previous one. During these times, I focused on being positive, continuing to do my healing and spiritual exercises. I went for a walk twice a day, in the morning and afternoon. I spoke to the plants and flowers, admiring them and praising their beauty. I expressed thanks that I still could walk and smell the roses. I listened to the birds chirping and pretended they were serenading me. I concentrated on shifting my focus from my suffering to the beauty of nature. In addition, I became more familiar with my neighborhood, talking with people who were walking their dogs or watering their gardens. I discovered an entire world around me that, until that point, I'd never known.

By this time, I wasn't afraid of the surgeries themselves anymore; I was afraid of their results. Mostly I wondered if the doctor was going to insert the implant in the correct position. After all, this was going to be my fourth surgery within four months, and the third surgery with the same doctor. I couldn't help but feel doubtful and afraid.

In addition, during one of these surgeries, the doctor reduced the size of my right breast to match the size of the implant on the left side. In between all these surgeries, the nurse also built a nipple on the implant. How ironic! They built a nipple on my flat left chest but not on the implant!

Next, I went through another surgery to remove the old implant and to insert a new one. I hoped that this time it could be placed in the right position on my chest. A few weeks after this surgery and after I had a saline injection, I felt the implant pulling downward on my chest. I called Dr. Pearson with panic in my voice and told him what I felt. He dismissed it, insisting that what I was feeling was normal. He suggested I put some duct tape below the implant to hold it up. *What a joke! A piece of duct tape would hold up the implant. What was the job of the surgeon, anyway? But what other choices did I have?* I followed his instructions and started using duct tape to hold it up. Unfortunately, I turned out to be allergic to the tape and couldn't use it. Once again, I began to panic. *Why was the implant going downward? Did it mean that it was not placed in the right spot again?* All my mistrust and worry became reality. In fact, on the next visit, my doctor agreed it had been placed too low on my chest.

This time, I became angrier than ever. After all, my doctors originally told me that this kind of surgery was a "piece of cake," a procedure done every day. *How could it be that easy if he didn't know exactly how or where to place the implant?* I tried to remain upbeat and smile, but in all honesty, I was furious.

My mastectomy nightmare was growing bigger every day. All I wanted was another breast so I could look at myself in the mirror and see my body whole again. It was easy for the doctor to say that he would simply do another surgery. For him it was routine, but for me it meant more misery.

Moreover, I found his unsympathetic tone annoying. Not only did he claim no responsibility for the mistakes he made, he also didn't act accountable or feel badly about putting me through another surgery and miserable recovery period. Although I knew on some level his mistakes weren't purposeful, I resented how awful I felt when I compared it to his nonchalance. His attitude, in fact, enraged me so much, I lost faith in him. *What was I to do now, entrust my body to him again?*

Whatever I decided, one thing was clear: at least one more surgery to remove the implant was in my future. Why? Because, my appearance with only one breast was unacceptable to me. My breasts had always been my pride and joy. As a single woman, I wondered how I would ever meet and be intimate with a man again. I worried that I wouldn't attract the kind of man who would want to have sexual relations with me, a woman who had only one breast. In addition, I couldn't face looking in the mirror and seeing only one breast. For these two reasons, I decided to undergo my fifth surgery in seven months, hoping the doctor would finally get it right.

A Vicious Cycle

This bad nightmare repeated itself like a vicious circle. Again, I had to find somebody to drive me to the hospital and pick me up. The pain of spending another day at the hospital and putting my body through anesthesia again was unbearable.

Thinking about it today, I don't know how I survived this part of my journey, but I went through the whole procedure again with great anticipation this would be the last time I had to place my body under the care of this doctor. Hallelujah! This implant was not on my belly, but was placed right where it was supposed to be. This called for celebration. I was finally going to have two breasts after all. I would be able to look in the mirror and see my whole body. I was ecstatic.

Sadly, my celebration was short-lived. I began suffering from constant pain and discomfort. During the next visit with Dr. Pearson, he told me the new implant was infected and sent me to the hospital for seven days for an antibiotic IV drip. He warned me that if the antibiotic did not clear up the infection, this implant would need to be removed. The antibiotic didn't clear the infection. The pain and agony continued. I'd reached the end of my rope.

Let Go and Let God

"Until you make peace with who you are, you'll never be content with what you have." — Doris Mortman

At this point, I had been fighting to have another breast for over half the year, with the only results being severe pain, emotional agony, fruitless anticipation, and utter disappointments. I needed to take back control over my life because I was unable to stand the treatments any longer.

Ultimately, I realized it was time to let go, to clear my mental, emotional, and physical space, to release my fears, worries, and disappointments, to put myself into the Universe's hands. I had to completely divorce myself from any emotional investment I had in reconstructing a new breast. My perspective on life had to change; I had to accept that having another breast wasn't important to me anymore.

"Too often we underestimate the power of a touch, a smile, a kind word, a listening ear, an honest compliment, or the smallest act of caring - all of which have the potential to turn a life around."
- Leo Buscaglia

CHAPTER 3

Taking Charge

"The Power that Heals is in the patient himself."
- Wallace D. Wattles

One morning, I woke up and called a friend and fellow patient, Diane, whom I had met during my IV drip treatment. I asked if she'd be willing to drive me to the hospital because, even though I didn't have an appointment, I was determined to have my failed implant removed *that* very day.

Diane and I went straight to the plastic surgery department and requested to see my surgeon. "Not available," I was told. I declared that "I'd had enough" and demanded the implant be removed that day. The nurse at the reception desk repeated the same monologue I'd just heard about my doctor being booked for other surgeries all day long. "And besides," she said, "you're not ready to have surgery today." I replied that, after having had five surgeries already, I knew the procedure. I also knew that I'd go crazy if the infected implant were not removed *that very day*. If my surgeon was booked, I insisted they find me another surgeon. I wouldn't leave the hospital until the implant was removed from my body. I adamantly refused to suffer one more day.

At this point, they realized they weren't going to get rid of me and my friend. So someone finally got my surgeon, Dr. Pearson, to come out and talk with me. He told me that if I waited until all of his other surgeries were completed, he would perform mine that evening between six and seven o'clock. Even though he said this at nine o'clock in the morning, I was willing to wait. I couldn't bear any more suffering.

I spent that entire day once again going though the procedure of signing papers and getting ready for another surgery, all with Diane at my side. May God bless her soul! She was very sick herself but at that time I didn't know how sick she was. She stayed to hold my hand and walk me through the getting-ready procedure.

As we sat in the waiting room to be called to go to the operating room for preparation, Diane still held my hand like a mother hen protecting her offspring. I knew she didn't have anything to eat that morning and that she needed to rest, so I told her to go home. Diane was adamant about staying and holding my hand, claiming that nobody should go through surgery alone. Although I told her I was used to it, deep down I was glad she was staying. Nonetheless, I insisted that she go home, have something to eat, get some rest, and return for me later. I went into surgery knowing that someone who cared about me would be there. I felt very grateful.

My Angel, Diane

To my delight, when I woke up from my surgery, I saw Diane immediately. Actually, she'd arrived at the hospital two hours before and had been waiting for me to wake up. In the past, friends who had picked me up at the hospital most often drove me home and left. This time, I knew I didn't want to be alone that night. Diane had been so supportive that I felt comfortable asking her if she'd stay overnight at my place. She replied, "I was hoping you would ask me that."

This beautiful being spent a whole day and a night with me during my sixth surgery. But it was more than her physical presence that counted; it was a rare but amazing feeling of intimacy, friendship and an unconditional love that I felt flowing from her soul to mine that made her my angel. I was in God's hands whenever I thought about her. Even though she couldn't do much physically, her vibration and devotion came to me so unselfishly, so generously, and at such a high level.

That night, Diane drove me home, fed me crackers, and gave me medication to help me sleep as she tucked me into bed like a child. At three o'clock in the morning, I woke up to noises coming from the living room where Diane was supposedly sleeping. The lights were on. I couldn't get out of bed, so I shouted out to Diane, "What's going on?" She said she had to go home because she couldn't breathe. Apparently, one of her illnesses was a breathing problem, which I hadn't known about. She had a breathing machine at home and needed to get to it as soon as possible. Despite her best intentions to take care of me, she urgently had to take care of herself.

Diane never said anything to make me feel guilty for the time and devotion she gave me that day. I appreciated her generosity of spirit and willingness to stay in touch by phone. Even today, not a day goes by that I'm not grateful for having her in my life during such a difficult time.

Later, I discovered so much more about Diane and how her acts of kindness proved to be angelic.

Diane did not have any family she'd lost her mother a few years earlier. A paralegal by profession, she was very bright. Unfortunately, due to her extensive medical problems—breast cancer, melanoma, and breathing problems—she hadn't been able to work much. She'd been engaged to be married but when her fiancé found out she had breast cancer, he broke off the engagement over the phone, telling her she "wasn't a woman anymore." She vowed never to speak to him again.

So in addition to cancer, Diane and I had another thing in common: we were both alone.

Over the following months, I attempted to support her, telling her all the things we would do together when she felt better. Then one day around Thanksgiving, I returned home after running errands and found a big box waiting for me behind the door. I assumed it had come to me by mistake. The sender's name, David Pears or something like that, wasn't familiar. Perhaps it came from my friends Bill and Sandra, who always used to throw big Thanksgiving parties and invite me. I had told very few people about my mastectomy, but because Bill and Sandra knew about it, I thought they'd sent the package to cheer me up.

Inside I found the most gorgeous fresh fruit and a card from the sender—my angel, Diane. I knew that she struggled to pay her own mortgage so I was especially amazed and touched by her kindness, yet embarrassed at the same time. I called her right away.

"Thanks so much. But, Diane, you should have used this money to pay your bills."

She replied, "You are a part of me, Lea! We are all ONE. I hope you enjoy the fruits."

Threads Woven into the Fabric of Life

Yes, I thought to myself, we are all ONE. Each person is a thread in a woven fabric of life and, together, we make a whole. Each thread has its own placement, its own path of integration, and its unique contribution to the unification of the fabric. I experienced this oneness and connectedness during my spiritual training; I also felt it when Diane had given of herself so selflessly at the time of my sixth surgery.

Unfortunately, I never had the chance to touch Diane the way she touched me. I'd call her often, but got her answering machine. I'd leave her multiple messages for her to call me back. When she didn't, I became concerned. My intuition told me she was home but wouldn't answer the phone. Later, I learned that talking made her out of breath, so she wouldn't pick up the phone unless it was an emergency.

One day I received a postcard from Diane. She wrote that I didn't understand the seriousness of her condition and that she no longer wanted to be in touch with me. So I respected her wishes and didn't contact her anymore. Still, my angel Diane was constantly on my mind.

When Christmas was approaching, I sent Diane a Christmas card. Two weeks later, I received a letter from a person I didn't know. It had Diane's return address on the envelope. *This is odd,* I thought and opened it with shaking hands. The letter inside was addressed to me by Claudia, one of her neighbors. She said that Diane had passed away about a month before. She enclosed a newspaper announcement of her death.

Claudia had kindly given me her phone number, so I called her immediately. I couldn't stop crying while listening to Claudia talk about Diane. I confided in her, telling her about my last contact with Diane and sharing how difficult it was for me to respect her wishes. Claudia told me Diane withdrew from all her friends because she didn't want them to worry about her, knowing her days on Earth were numbered.

What a special being, this angel who appeared in my life when I most needed someone to lean on. She disappeared from my life like an angel, too, to spare me the agony of her death. If I didn't believe in angels before, Diane's appearance proved that angels do exist. Naturally, I became a believer. She enriched my life in so many ways—one of the threads of the fabric that makes me feel connected. My angel, Diane, you will be in my heart forever!

CHAPTER 4

No Longer Feeling All Alone

"When we feel love and kindness toward others, it not only makes others feel loved and cared for, but it helps us also to develop inner happiness and peace."
— The Dalai Lama

If I felt alone during my battle with cancer, I didn't feel alone once I discovered weSPARK, a non-profit cancer support center within walking distance of my home in Sherman Oaks, California. This is another amazing story of how things manifest in our lives when we need them the most. I was going to a yoga class for cancer patients at St. Joseph's Hospital, when somebody handed me a brochure about weSPARK. One day during my daily walk, I decided to stop by and find out what it was all about. It was in the fall of 2001 when they had just opened the doors to the public.

weSPARK was founded by Wendie Jo Sperber, an actress and comedian who exuded energy and made living life with cancer bearable. Although she was small in stature, no dream was too big for Wendie Jo. When she had been diagnosed with breast cancer eight years earlier, she sought support and found her options lacking. Determined to help herself and others, her devotion and giving spirit drove her to create weSPARK. Wendie Jo's presence inspired everyone at the support center every day. Never complaining about her own condition, she supervised activities and encouraged all the "guests" to never give up.

The center provides services free of charge to anyone who either has cancer or is a relative and/or caretaker for someone with this illness. It organizes several support groups as well as classes in yoga, guided imagery, energy work, Qi Gong, Tai Chi, and others. Staff members are devoted individuals eager to help people during their wrenching cancer journeys. (Go to Appendix B to learn more about this vital non-profit support group and get involved, too!)

Once the word about weSPARK got out, volunteers kept coming, some contributing financially and others giving of their time. Their generous actions were heartily received by people affected by cancer.

Finding Sanctuary

Peace and tranquility embraced me not only when I first walked through the doorway but every time I visited weSPARK. The center became my sanctuary, a home away from home, a warm, cozy, place that, upon entering, people feel like they're being invited into somebody's living room to share tea and biscuits on a rainy afternoon. I spent many hours at weSPARK taking classes and giving seminars about spirituality and personal growth. I talked with other guests and listened to stories about their battles with cancer.

I owe tremendous gratitude to Wendie Jo, her staff, and all the volunteers who made my road to recovery more bearable in this haven. Wendie Jo's contagious driving spirit greatly influenced my personal growth and development. I learned from her that everything is possible. Indeed, this book would not have been written without her influence; therefore, the book is dedicated to her and the center that nourishes so many people during their darkest moments. Most importantly, thanks to weSPARK, I no longer felt isolated. To Wendie Jo, who left this planet in November 2005, may she know that the legacy of her mission is invaluable to cancer survivors like myself.

"Make it a rule of life never to regret and never to look back. Regret is an appalling waste of energy; you can't build on it; it's only for wallowing in."
- Katherine Mansfield

CHAPTER 5

Self-Acceptance

"Be the change you want to see in the world."
— Mahatma Gandhi

During my illness and recovery, I had met many women with breast cancer and who were ashamed of their bodies and believed they'd lost their femininity. They were afraid, worried that no men would be sexually attracted to them anymore. That's exactly what I felt at the beginning of my arduous breast cancer journey.

Accepting the fact that I had to live with one breast was traumatic.

There are no manuals or books that one can purchase and follow the instructions to get over this incredible trauma that so many women have to face. Surgeons know how to surgically remove the breast, but psychologists are at a loss about how to mend the emotional incision cancer makes in our lives. The only other option that I could see was to work on myself from the spiritual aspect. So far, I had concentrated completely on my physical appearance which I fought to regain.

However, when I approached the situation on a spiritual level, I realized that I am the same whole woman. Lack of one breast did not have that kind of impact on my existence of being a whole woman. True, it's not esthetic when I look in the mirror, but does it make me less of a woman? NO! I am the same woman who went through a trauma that in the end enriched my life. I became a better person and learned a crucial life lesson. I inventoried my situation again, focusing on what I gained from this experience rather than what I lost.

When I reached that state of mind, I realized how many more women go through what I went through, and how I might help them to feel like whole women again.

My sole purpose became to create more awareness that we are not only a body. We are spirit with a soul that functions through our body. I made it my mission to assist other women crippled by any notion that they've lost their femininity.

As an example, I had met a psychologist, a professional woman who had breast cancer and successfully had an implant done. When I met her, I wondered why she was wearing a scarf around her neck during the scorching heat of the Los Angeles summer. Then one day I discovered that, in her mind's eye, one of her breasts seemed smaller than the other. To cover up the smaller one, she always wore a scarf.

Some breast cancer survivors never recover from fears like this. My heart goes out to them when they can't overcome fears of being sexually undesirable to men after their mastectomies. Some of them see themselves as victims of this disease. Some were even unable to admit they had breast cancer because they consider it such a stigma.

I became determined to be "the change I wanted to see" in the world of women breast cancer survivors. I repurposed Gandhi's profound advice as "What can I do to change what I want to see among women survivors of breast cancer?"

Gandhi also said: *"Loving what you hate sends a positive, beautiful energy to people while spreading peace and harmony throughout the planet. Instead of reinforcing hatred, you become an advocate for love. Hatred responds to hate by causing anguish. However, love responds to hatred by transforming it into blissful peace."*

I have made that concept my life's agenda—to advocate loving our bodies after mastectomy. We don't need to be ashamed or fearful about how society may react or perceive us.

Baring My Soul's Purpose

Yes, I had a burning desire to transform the hatred of my new image into blissful peace—mentally, physically, and spiritually. And I constantly wondered how I could help other women change their minds and attitudes about their sexuality and intimacy with men.

How could I influence them to be able to look at themselves as whole women with one breast or even with no breasts? How could I awaken their inner spirits and expose them to spiritual enlightenment?

It's amazing what opportunities present themselves when a person has clear intentions and a mindset to accomplish what the heart desires. Here's what happened for me at the perfect moment.

Three years after my mastectomy, I attended a three-day seminar to sharpen my public speaking skills and learn how to deliver seminars. Our schedule started at 9:00 a.m. and continued until midnight. The curriculum consisted of various experiential exercises and lecture.

The first day of the seminar, I learned that all the participants were expected to get on stage and do something outrageous for ninety seconds in front of three hundred and fifty perfect strangers. The purpose was to allow them to free themselves of their inhibitions.

Apparently, an email had been sent to everyone about this requirement, but for some reason—either I didn't receive the email or I didn't read it thoroughly—I wasn't aware of it. The email also told participants to bring their own music, costumes, props, or whatever they needed for their outrageous presentations.

I hadn't brought anything with me. Still, I had to decide what I'd do when my turn came. Then I heard an announcement: extra props could be taken from a table set up for this purpose. Yes, that would solve my problem. By the time I approached the table, only these props were left: a pair of silver lamé pants, a gold lamé top, and six Hawaiian leis in different lengths. I picked them up, trusting that these items would be *perfect* for what I intended to do on stage.

Most participants had brought elaborate costumes and the right music for their outrageous performances. One woman dressed as an opera singer and sang an aria. Another who was dressed to the hilt dropped her top and flashed her bare breasts during her performance. One gent dressed as Elvis Presley mimicked Elvis's singing. Others showed off their talents as comedians while several danced or sang on stage.

I had a different idea completely.

My turn to appear on stage was to fall on the second evening, so on the first evening, I watched the others perform. When one woman played "Day by Day," a top 1960s hit by the Fifth Dimension, I thought, *"this song would be a perfect match for my act."* So I asked to borrow her music and she agreed.

The next evening before the performances started, I debated if I should go ahead and use my new-found props to be truly outrageous on stage, too. My head was spinning, my heart was pounding: *kaboom, kaboom.* So I closed my eyes and placed both hands on my heart. I breathed deeply and let my spiritual exercises calm me down. Finally, I reached a state of peace and calmness. Then I knew. *I was on a mission.* I got up and donned my costume. I placed two of the small leis around my two upper arms, one bigger size around my head, and three of the longer sizes around my neck, layered a sweater over top, and walked backstage to the performance room.

My Mission Revealed On Stage

"When we are motivated by goals that have deep meaning, by dreams that need completion, by pure love that needs expressing, then we truly live life."
— Greg Anderson

Before long, it was my turn. Like the others, I had to put on a headset with a microphone. As the stage hands fit it on my head, one girl whispered in my ear, "You will be great. They will love you." I replied, "Yes, I know. I want to make a powerful statement."

The chosen musical selection began to play and I danced with it while singing the words of "Day by Day." Then I turned my back to the audience, stripped off my gold lamé top, and turned around to face the people. I threw my top into the audience. They couldn't see much of my chest because I still had the Hawaiian leis around my neck. Then I took off the leis and threw them one by one into the crowd. By this time, they could clearly see that I had only one breast. They cheered and clapped their hands exuberantly.

I was on stage only ninety seconds. When the music ended, I ran off covering myself with both my hands. Someone in the front handed me my sweater and pushed me back on stage to take a bow. Going wild, people were standing up, cheering and clapping as if I were a celebrity at a concert.

During those ninety seconds I didn't feel like it was *my* body on that stage. I felt like I was on a different planet, not acting, but being the real me. I felt a strong connection to the Source, to my core being. I felt connected to my pure spirit, using my body as a vehicle that let me demonstrate my whole being. In that moment, I totally accepted my body just the way it was. No shame or embarrassment. Egoless. Pure. I had exposed my soul to make a powerful statement.

People in the audience picked up on the authenticity of my act, which is exactly what I intended. I also wanted to convey awareness about breast cancer and about women who after their mastectomies live in fear of intimacy and rejection by men. As I exited the stage, they lined up to give me hugs, cry with me, laugh with me, and tell me how courageous I was. I heard whispering voices say "Thank you! Thank you!" multiple times. And I heard one person say, "You cannot imagine what you did for the sake of women in the same situation."

I felt fully connected with them. I firmly believe they embraced me because I had accepted my new

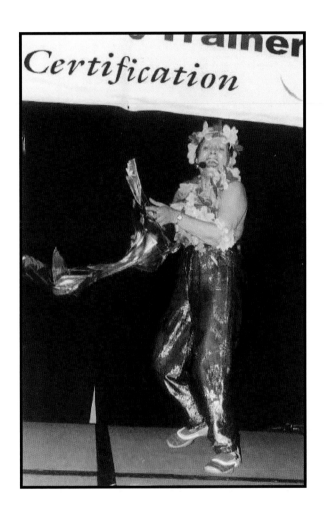

90-second performance on stage - 2003

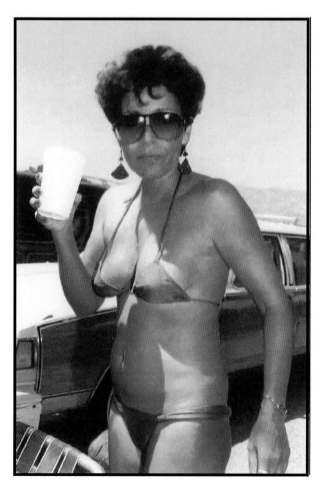

Lea on vacation

image internally and spiritually, in my True Spirit. This simple action of exposing my imperfection in front of three hundred and fifty strangers gave them the courage and permission to admit their own flaws—to be imperfect themselves, physically and otherwise. More than that, in projecting an image of a person who exuded self-confidence, independence, and sexual security, not only did I bring awareness to women in the same situation; I believe I also helped men realize that women with one breast could be attractive and desirable.

Even at the end of the seminar, both men and women kept approaching me to hug me and thank me for being myself. Among them were doctors who specialized in cancer treatments. They handed me their business cards, probably thinking they could help me. No, thanks. I've already traveled along that route.

How the Universe Delivers

Perhaps you wondered about the answers to these questions as I did after this experience.

- Was it an accident I didn't receive that email about the performances or didn't read it thoroughly?

- Do you think it was coincidence or luck that I easily found all the props I needed on the table?

- Why was I the one who approached the table last?

- How can anybody explain that the remaining props were perfect for what I wanted to convey on stage?

- How is it possible that those props were the only items left on the table and nothing else?

The answer to all the above questions is the "Law of Attraction."

Law of Attraction

The Law of Attraction is a simple universal law. Its tenets are:

1. Like attracts like.

2. What you focus on expands.

3. When your conscious and subconscious mind are in harmony to accomplish anything your heart desires, the universe will collaborate totally with your wishes and bring them into manifestation.

4. Everything is created through energetic vibration. Sound is vibration. Light is vibration. Thought is vibration. Emotion is vibration. Everything is vibration. Anything that vibrates at a specific rate will attract similar vibrations. This works on the, physical, mental, emotional and spiritual level.

5. Good or bad, you always attract what you think about.

Now, you can see how the Universe was collaborating with my thoughts. It picked up on the vibrations that I was sending out, that I wanted to create more awareness about spirituality and empower women who feel sexually undesirable to men.

The Universe arranged this experience perfectly so I could fulfill my mission. It works in mysterious ways—ways that our naked eyes simply cannot see!

The Source of Fear of Intimacy

The word 'intimacy' is defined by various dictionaries as: "affection, caring, close relationship, confidentiality, friendship, companionship, affinity, and sexual relation."

As you can tell, there are many different definitions for the word and perhaps you realize that there is a subtle thread which weaves a commonality among such varied definitions. That common quality implicit in all of the above is trust.

I trusted that perfect strangers would accept me as I bared my breasts. The audience's reaction to my performance indicated that I made some personal impact by doing so and a more global one by bringing the issue of mastectomy into the open. Their reaction also told me how taboo the subject was to talk about; perhaps that's exactly why it needed to be talked about. No one approached me and asked me for a date (that was not my intention) but I did cause quite a stir. Yes, that audience was receptive and welcomed the subject. But I was curious to find out what happens when people face this issue on a one-on-one basis. What would be a man's reaction when faced with the difficult reality of living with a woman with one breast or none?

After my life-changing performance, I did extensive research by talking with hundreds of men to get their views on this issue. Some men emailed me their opinion and some just told me verbally. According to the feedback I received, the reactions were divided into three types:

A. Fearful. The men who were never exposed to the world of cancer and especially breast cancer and mastectomy, often expressed fear and they did not know what their reaction would be if their own significant other had breast cancer or a mastectomy. They worried how the situation would affect their sexual life. Mostly, they feared the unknown. They could not even imagine encountering a situation like that.

B. Very reserved. They hesitated to express their opinion. These men had encountered medical situations like this, but were not willing to talk about their feelings.

C. Very open about it. These men had experienced breast cancer and its effects first-hand or knew of a friend or a family member who were affected by this disease. They were scared at the beginning but they overcame it when they learned more about it.

This whole situation of fear of intimacy after mastectomy and the different reactions about it haunted me. I needed to know men's perspectives when they heard that a woman had breast cancer or a mastectomy.

I decided to meditate about it in order to find answers to this complicated issue. For about two weeks, I meditated daily for hours, waiting for enlightenment on how to find the information. As the saying goes: "When the student is ready the master appears." And indeed he did appear in my life, out of nowhere. He was a wise and open-minded man who was willing and could talk frankly with me. I took with me my tape recorder to our nearby coffee shop where we met. I was blessed to meet him and had the opportunity to discuss this issue with him. When I told him of my quest to understand how men perceive mastectomy, the conversation went on for hours.

"Lea", he asked; "have you ever gone snorkeling?"

"Of course, I love snorkeling. Especially in Mexico where the water in the ocean is so clear and I can see all kinds of fish with different colors, shapes and sizes."

"Do you know that all of the ocean inhabitants have their own likes and dislikes, have their own characteristics?"

"Yes," I said.

"You see, Lea, if the fish in the ocean have certain characteristics, have their likes and dislikes, so do human beings. Each person may react differently to the same circumstance because of their background and what experiences they had gone through in their many lives."

"Ok, I understand that part," I said. "But why does a woman's breast have such an impact on men? Why is it so hard for some men to be open to intimacy with women who have one breast or none?" I was eager to learn how a man's mind works.

He told me that when men hear that a woman had breast cancer or a mastectomy, these are the things they think about:

1.   If she lost her breast, they think she lost her femininity at the same time and, therefore, she is not a woman anymore.

2.   And if she is not a woman anymore, obviously she has lost her sexual desire.

3.   Therefore, they are not attracted to her anymore.

4.   They develop fear of not being able to have the option of foreplay before love-making.

5.   They think that a woman's breasts are what make her a woman and if she had lost one due to a mastectomy, she is not a woman anymore.

6.   They know if they lost their own penis they would not be able to have a sexual relationship. They feel it's the same situation with a woman if she lost her breast.

7.   All these misconceptions stem from the fear of the unknown.

Here is an example of a man named Eric, who I spoke with on the phone. He is a married man and author by profession. He writes about "Love and Relationships." He admitted to me that the thought of cancer scares him to death! He cannot even imagine how he would react toward his wife if the disease were to hit home.

The above list typically applies to type "A" men.

Negative Reactions from Men

For instance I know a married couple, Joanna and David by name. David could not even look at Joanna's chest, let alone have an intimate relationship after she had a mastectomy on one breast.
The following is an email I received from Laura, a woman who had a double mastectomy.

I was in my late forties and married for fifteen years to the same man when I was diagnosed with breast cancer. The doctors recommended double mastectomy. They thought it was the best solution for my situation at the time. My marriage was not perfect to begin with and the double mastectomy added more problems to my marriage. Instead of supporting me, my husband then had more reasons to keep us apart. He refused to have any intimacy with me. He found another woman and I knew about her. I felt devastated and humiliated emotionally as well as physically. But I was scared to death to confront him about it or divorce him. I thought if my husband of fifteen years rejected me because of my double mastectomy, what other man would want to have any relationship with me? After four years of living in hell and misery I could not take it anymore, I reached the end of my rope and recently I got divorced.

Even though I live alone, I am sorry I did not divorce him earlier. Now, at least I have my dignity. Of course, I still live with the fear that no man would want to have any relationship with me. The truth is that I don't even know how to mingle with people, since my self-esteem is so low after being in that relationship for such a long time.

I am familiar with another case of a couple named Edna and Jonathan; they lived together. As soon as she was diagnosed with breast cancer, he immediately broke up with her—a story that echoes the case of Diane in the earlier chapter. Her fiancé did not even have the courage or decency to communicate his decision in person: he broke their engagement on the phone.

Type "B" men tend to have these fears:

1.   They think that if the woman had a mastectomy, she may have some emotional problems coping with it.

2.   They have the fear of recurrence.

3.   Or maybe one day she may collapse on them.

Stories of Unconditional Love for Women After Mastectomy

Not all men are afraid. When I met Linda she was in her mid-sixties and had a double mastectomy thirty years earlier. A man fell in love with her and it did not matter to him at all that she did not have breasts.

I know another married couple, Jim and Mary. After her mastectomy, whenever she put on a bathing suit, her husband insisted that she wear a bikini and put a prosthesis inside her bra to look beautiful and sexy in public, so other people could notice her beauty even after mastectomy.

This couple's story is extraordinary. Deborah was a breast cancer survivor who was also the founder of the Cancer Support Center. Located next to the Cancer Support Center was a small gym. One day she walked to the gym, accompanied by a twelve year-old boy with cancer. She asked the facility owner if he would train the boy at no charge. "The moment Deborah walked into my gym with that boy, my life totally changed" he told me. He agreed to train the youngster with cancer at no charge. Soon after, he found himself helping the Cancer Support Center in any way he possibly could. He invited all the cancer patients at that cancer support center to use his gym at no charge. He even designed special classes for cancer survivors. He eventually fell in love with Deborah. Their relationship became so close, they were a team, and found themselves physically attracted to each other in spite of her mastectomy.

Here is an email I received from Susan.

When I was diagnosed with breast cancer and had a mastectomy to remove one breast, I was in my mid-twenties and happily married. My husband was very supportive all the way. I did not even attempt a breast implant. With the support of my husband, I became a breast cancer activist. The only concern we had was that I may not be able to get pregnant because of the chemo and radiation treatment I had.

We decided to adopt a child. Sure enough, after the adoption I discovered that I was pregnant. Now, we have two beautiful children six months apart in age from each other.

Debby told me another amazing story of her husband's love when she was diagnosed with breast cancer. Her husband was the sole caregiver and supported her 100%. He went with her to all the doctors' appointments, and accompanied her to her chemo treatments. He even wrote a book entitled "Cancer for Two." The title of his book speaks for itself. This couple exemplifies that a solid foundation of intimacy in the sense of friendship must also form the basis of sexual intimacy.

These men are all type "C" men.

My Own Experiences

From my own experience, I had a relationship with a man right after my last implant was removed and while I was in the recovery period. He knew vaguely about my condition since we were members of the same organization. However, when I felt that the relationship was turning more serious, I asked him if he knew about my condition. He said "yes," and that it did not matter to him at all. Eventually, he even asked me to marry him.

Here is another experience I had. A man contacted me via the Internet. We communicated for a while through email and phone calls, but I never met him in person. In one of our communications I decided to reveal more about myself. I figured if this relationship was going to continue any further, I might as well tell him about my condition. Since I have an ebook with articles about self- improvement and spiritual growth, I sent him the link to the ebook, so he could read and learn more about me. In the ebook was also my bio that indicated, among other things, that I was a cancer survivor. After this communication, I did not hear from him again.

One day about five weeks later, I received a phone call from him. He was in town and invited me out for dinner, which I agreed to without any hesitation.

During dinner, I asked him what made him decide to call me after he stopped emailing me. His answer was that he felt "guilty" because he was touched by one of my articles entitled the "Power of Forgiveness." He also told me that he never met a woman with breast cancer and my bluntness about it caught him off guard. It was obvious that we were not a good match.

As part of the research for this book, I sent him an email requesting that he express his honest feelings when he read about my condition. Here is his response in his own words.

As for you and me, I did not walk away from you because of your breast cancer: that, for me, was not an issue. You were very open and I liked that. It did not upset me in any way that you had breast cancer. That is just one of those things. I was curious [as to] how you dealt with it sexually and as a person. As a person, I can remember thinking how open you were. I thought that was very refreshing. How you dealt with it sexually I never found out. There is no question that breasts are important for different reasons for both men and women. From a sexual point of view, I think a woman can help herself and her partner by being open and by counteracting the lack of breasts by emphasizing other sexual attributes and making sure that she is comfortable with herself. If she is comfortable with her situation, then the man should feel at ease. I know myself the fact that you were so open about your situation made me feel very comfortable (about the fact) that you did not have both your breasts.

I posed the same question to a man who was in a long-time relationship with his girlfriend with whom he was living. He wrote his response.

If my long-time girlfriend had a mastectomy, it would make no difference to me.

If I find out that another woman who was not ever going to be a love interest of mine had a mastectomy, again it would make no difference to me.

If I found out that a potential love interest had a mastectomy before we had any kind of significant relationship, I would be hesitant to take the romantic relationship too far. Reason is that I would worry, that she might relapse and die on me, and also that she may be having significant emotional problems with the mastectomy that no amount of patience on my part could overcome her state of mind.

Here is another reaction of a man who took so much of his time to email me his feelings. Read his detailed response.

If my wife had a mastectomy:
I would remain intimate with her as before. I would find out if there are any 'sensitive' or painful areas on her chest so as not to give her any pain or discomfort. I would kiss and caress the area of the surgery and assure my wife that the loss of a breast(s) does not mean the loss of my love or how I perceive her. I would assure her that breasts are for child rearing i.e., to let newborns suckle from. If she never breast fed, then I would still tell my wife how much I deeply love her now, as before, and that nothing would change that. I would tell my wife that I married her for her heart and soul, and not for her body.

If my girlfriend had a mastectomy:
As with my wife, I would assure my girlfriend that I love her for who she is, not who she appears to be cosmetically. I would assure my girlfriend that despite the allure of breasts to some men, the absence of a breast(s) does not make her ugly, deformed, or incomplete. I would love my girlfriend spiritually and physically in order to show her that my love for her comes from my heart and not my penis.

If I were single [and] seeking a significant other:
I would remain open-minded. The absence of a breast(s) would not have any impact on me; i.e., I would seek a mature, interesting, funny, and curious person to date–and perhaps marry. If I found a woman

who had a mastectomy, I would not see her as anything other than a complete person. Complete defined as being equal to any other woman. The absence of a breast(s) does not take anything away from the woman that has come to accept this situation and approaches it with a realistic, mature, attitude. I would still seek out the woman for her love, her mind, her heart, her funny little quirks that make up her character. I would calm her fears and assure her that I love her as a person and not as a complete set of breasts. I would not let this condition interfere with my intimacy with her.

If nothing else, I would be even more intimate in all three situations (above) as I would love this woman for being so brave, so proud, and so strong. This would be a 'turn on' to me as I would not love her out of pity, but out of the knowledge that she is a survivor and undoubtedly the stronger person between us two.

The bottom line is that women after undergoing a radical procedure that removes one or both breasts will undoubtedly become withdrawn and introverted. This is vanity that we all possess. Accepting one's condition and dealing with it on a daily basis makes these women stronger in the long run. Do we love a war hero any less when he returns missing limbs or sight?

Women who survive a cancer that takes away the symbol of womanhood from them are stronger people in the end. Of course this is my opinion, speaking as a man that has not undergone the rigors of a breast removal. Men should never assume that a woman who has had a mastectomy is somewhat less than whole. A woman's breasts are beautiful appendages that signal to a man the femininity of the woman. However, breasts are largely organs that have ensured the survival of the species in all mammals. If men cease to understand the purpose of breasts and become fixated with the titillating prospects of feeling and caressing them for no other reason than to have intercourse, is at best predictable male behavior and juvenile.

That some men would be repulsed or 'turned off' by a woman bearing both the mental and physical scars of a mastectomy would define a very shallow and ignorant individual. There are men such as myself that would embrace figuratively and literally a woman for who she is, not who she feels that society wants her to be. I would love any woman, with breasts or none, who would have me and accept me as a person and not as a sex symbol. I would feel honored to find someone like this. By the same token, I would give my heart and soul to any woman who would reciprocate equally the love and affection that I give her.

Well, in my opinion he is the men's MAN. Wouldn't you just love to have a man like this in your life?

"Any person capable of angering you becomes your master; he can anger you only when you permit yourself to be disturbed by him."
- Epictetus

CHAPTER 6

Knowledge Is Power

"You can conquer almost any fear if you will only make up your mind to do so. For remember, fear doesn't exist anywhere except in the mind." -Dale Carnegie

One of humankind's greatest fears is fear of the unknown. Once I began to learn more about breast cancer, I was able to make better decisions about my treatment. Similarly, after this research, I had a better idea of the male perspective on mastectomies. Since the best way to deal with fear is to understand, I wondered what would be the best way to help men understand so I asked my male friend.

"OK", I said, "Now as a woman who had a mastectomy, I would like to have a better understanding of the issue from a man's point of view. But we know that some of the men's concerns are not valid. What can women do to bridge the gap about this issue?"

He looked at me very thoughtfully and said, "The notion that men are stronger than women is just a fallacy that men created. Also, you can't change people unless they are willing to change. In order to bridge the gap, women have to educate themselves first. By educating themselves first, they will be able to educate men."

"How do you propose it should be done?" I asked.

"Lea," he said, "the acronym of fear is False Evidence Appearing Real."

As a rule of thumb, fear stems from anything that is unknown and misunderstood. If men are kept in the dark because women are afraid to open up and talk about it, women will keep experiencing rejection.

I realized then that the rejection women feel does not come from men; it comes from within themselves. Here is a quote from *A Course in Miracles*: "Perception is a mirror, not a fact. What I see is my state of mind, reflected outward."

Let's put it this way. If you look in the mirror, what do you see? You see your own reflection in the mirror. If there is fear, lack of confidence or low self-esteem in your reflection, it's all negative energy. If you feel and vibrate negative energy about yourself, it's automatically transmitted and projected to men. As a result, you will get a negative response from men.

"Energy goes where vibration flows." The healing process has to be initiated first by women themselves through their inner spirit. Women have to tap into their own natural power. Healing is the result of a person's consciousness guiding her life forces in the right direction.

As women, we have to do a lot of work on ourselves before we can educate and enlighten the men in our lives.

Let us:

1. Look at ourselves on a spiritual level, by fully accepting and owning our condition.

2. Know in our heart that our sexuality does not depend on having one breast or two breasts.

3. Realize that we are not our breasts. We are still whole women, even with only one breast.

4. Accept that now is the beginning of our new life. Appreciate our new life and enjoy every moment of it.

5. Celebrate our lives even with one breast or none.

6. Reclaim our femininity after mastectomy.

7. Rebuild our confidence living with one breast.

8. Accept our new image and love it.

9. Realize that fear of intimacy is in our own head and we have the power to change it.

10. Appreciate that sexuality exudes from inside out and not from outside in.

11. Transform our love lives from the state of fear and rejection to a state of openness, joy, acceptance and feeling whole as women.

When we accept ourselves, when we acknowledge ourselves, appreciate ourselves, approve of ourselves, count our blessings with grace and gratitude, just the way we are with one breast or none, miracles will happen in our lives.

When we honor ourselves, are kind to ourselves, love ourselves with optimism and passion, we create a positive perception and positive thinking, enjoy the here and now at the present moment; our cups always overflow.

When we feel good about ourselves, approach life with a joyful state of mind, embrace our new image as whole women, talk about it openly at an appropriate time with men who show interest in us, we make ourselves available for intimacy. When we speak about our breast at an appropriate time, we show vulnerability and feelings. All these feelings will lead us to the state of mind of allowing the right man to appear in our lives. Showing vulnerability is not weakness. It is a way to ignite good feelings, to get in touch with our spirit, and accept our unique selves. We can create positive intimacy with our loved ones by being ourselves and educating ourselves first. All the fear and misconception have a better chance of being cleared if we intimately know ourselves.

Some men may still be scared of having any relationship with you, but this is their problem not yours. On the other hand, some men may develop great respect and appreciation to your openness and courage and fall in love with YOU. A missing breast won't make any difference to them. Men will perceive what we project and vibrate. If we project and vibrate confidence, courage, independence and wholesomeness, that's how men will perceive us. So it's time to clean up our own act in order to create the proper awareness among the men in our lives.

I encountered many women who had breast cancer or a mastectomy and who would never talk about it out of fear about how other people might react. There is such a misunderstanding about cancer. There are cultures that do not even use the word "cancer" when someone is diagnosed. They call it a "difficult disease", as if it were a contagious disease or some kind of plague. There are other people who equate cancer with a death sentence.

There is no magic bullet answer to this complex situation. But, surely, hiding ourselves is not the answer. I overcame this fear because I recognized that I am not only my body. I am a spirit—that's the real me—that functions through my body. I am not defined by my breast. I learned this from my own experience, through the research I had done and from people who have talked to me.

How can women reach a more holistic state of mind?

In order to reach such a state of mind, we first have to understand how the conscious and subconscious aspects of our mind work. When we have that understanding, it's much easier to gain better control over our minds. When we have that understanding, we gain better control over our feelings and learn how to better direct our vibration to people and places.

How Our Conscious Mind Operates

"The mind is like a monkey swinging from branch to branch through the forest. In order not to lose sight of the monkey, we must watch the monkey constantly and even be one with it."
— Thich Nhat Hanh

Each of us has a conscious mind and a subconscious mind. Generally speaking, it is the nature of our conscious mind to be literal, rational, logical, serious, and negative. It tends to resist positive messages, such as "I am loveable," especially when you feel less than a whole woman at the moment. You may not even be aware of thoughts such as: "You will never be a whole woman again." No matter how much you try to reprogram these negative messages on a conscious level, the emotional imprints are so deep that negative beliefs will prevail.

Our conscious mind uses common sense, analyzes the information it receives, and organizes it into a logical framework. It goes into a mode of trying to "figure out" every thought, idea, or any creation we come up with. Sometimes these functions of our conscious mind are helpful; other times they can sabotage our dreams, stopping them from being fulfilled. Our conscious mind is a source of doubt and has a negative mental attitude.

Our subconscious mind, on the other hand, is a source of faith and has a positive mental attitude. This is not to say that one is bad and the other is good; that one is right and the other is wrong. It is a healthy dialogue between these ongoing in our mind that encourages us to make progress tempered with caution. Being more aware of how we think, we can learn how to use our brains more effectively. It is as if there are countless rooms in the mansion of our mind. Some are lavishly appointed and others quite sparse. Some of the rooms make us feel frightened, or angry, or resentful the moment we enter. In other rooms, there is energy teeming with creativity that draws us up into action. There are rooms that inspire hope and foster new relationships, and others filled with memories of what has already come to pass, and of other dreams that never did. Most people think they find themselves at any given point in a day in one room or another, without ever realizing that every second of every day, they consciously choose in which room to hang out. The more time we spend in any given room, gazing from its windows, the more the outside world begins to justify, reinforce, and, in every case, resemble it.

How Our Subconscious Mind Works

"The intuitive mind is a sacred gift and the rational mind is a faithful servant. We have created a society that honors the servant and has forgotten the gift." - Albert Einstein

It has been proven over the last fifty years through many studies and reports that the subconscious mind is able to absorb information that the conscious mind does not focus on or ignores. In fact, in many cases, it can absorb more when it does not focus on it! It is opposite to what one would naturally think.

Napoleon Hill told us almost seventy years ago that "any impulse of thought which is repeatedly passed on to the subconscious mind is finally accepted and acted upon by the subconscious mind, which proceeds to translate that impulse into its physical equivalent by the most practical process available." He recognized the power of the subconscious so much that he devoted an entire chapter to it in his book *Think and Grow Rich*.

"The subconscious mind will transmute into its physical equivalent, by the most direct and practical media available, any order which is given to it in a state of belief, or faith that the order will be carried out."

The nature of our subconscious mind is to be more positive, playful, and visual. The creative, intuitive mind is less discriminating. It absorbs information without question or analysis. It simply doesn't have the capacity of calculation.

Let's go back to the concept of the thought being a seed, because it is imperative to clearly understand the importance of what actually transpires in our mind as cancer survivors or women who have undergone mastectomy. Every thought is a seed at the conceptual level. When a seed is planted in fertile soil (feelings already established) this seed (thought/feeling) will then—create a reaction to that thought/feeling, or create the physical expression of that thought/feeling.

Now we have, as it is commonly known, an emotion. This emotion then becomes a living vibration, which fertilizes that seed/soil (thought/feeling), and we begin to grow our crop of effects (conditions in our life). In other words, thoughts and feelings create an emotion that causes effects.

Are you with me?

Any word or piece of data chosen by our conscious mind establishes images within our subconscious mind. If we think in a positive manner, visualize what we want, and dare to dream, we will get whatever we want.

It is that simple!

The Conflict

Let's face it—from time to time most of us feel that life is just one big struggle with a series of never-ending problems. In my case, it was breast cancer and mastectomy.

Yet, the truth is that life does not have to be this way. In fact, it can be just the opposite. Life is not about struggle and overcoming problems. Life is about pursuing and creating what we truly desire in an easy, stress-free manner.

In short, if you don't have what you want (you name it) your subconscious holds some contradictory intentions for you. To put it simply, you want something and it doesn't. For example, you may say subconsciously: "I want to be healthy, free of cancer" but your conscious belief may be, "Who am I kidding?" I have breast cancer; therefore, life is a struggle."

Do you notice anything different about these two statements? They are going in different directions. They are not in harmony. What is critical to understand is the competition, confliction agendas and disharmony between your conscious and subconscious mind that is preventing you from keeping positive thoughts and positive vibrations. Why? Because, when your conscious and subconscious are in disagreement, they produce negative emotion. And it is that very negative emotion or energy that attracts the things you don't want.

What does this mean for you? This means that once you figure out how to hold your conscious and subconscious mind in harmony, you will be in control of your life.

Change Your Attitude, Change Your Life

We human beings are in total control of the emotions that come into our mind and influence our thoughts and actions. More importantly, we can close the door to certain feelings and open it for others. We can develop the ability to channel the energy of our feelings to manifest in a positive way. We may let our cancer control us and rule our life, or we may chose to control our cancer by accepting it, owning it. How can we accept it? By practicing these actions:

1. Being aware of the feelings that pass through our consciousness.

2. Acknowledging our power over the circumstances.

3. Tapping into a desire to let in only positive feelings instead of negative ones.

4. Being willing to change so we can develop our ability to replace the negative with the positive, knowing it leads to a life of happiness and fulfillment.

Evoking positive feelings changes our inner attitude and influences our subconscious mind as well as our habits, actions, and reactions. As the driving force behind thoughts, feelings have great power. Thoughts without feelings are weak, but when they're energized by feelings, they become a mighty force.

Feelings drive actions that can be constructive or destructive, depending on whether our feelings are positive or negative. If we let positive feelings inspire and motivate us, we experience a great power that can improve our health and other aspects of our lives.

Think about your life for a moment and ask these questions:

1. When do you have the desire to act?

2. When are you able to get things done? (Is it when you have leisurely thoughts or when you're stirred by strong feelings?)

3. How do you act when you're incited by anger?

4. How do you act when you're irritated?

5. How do you act when you're inspired by strong love?

6. How do you act when you're feeling ambitious?

Understandably, it's not easy to drive away negative feelings if they have always ruled your life. People sometimes get so used to their habitual pessimistic feelings that even when they recognize how detrimental they are, they find it hard to stop them. This may sound strange, but it's possible to get used to bad habits and become attached to them, even knowing it's better to live without them. These habits can include constant worry about your condition.

Try this exercise.

---

1. Close your eyes and imagine a situation in which you experienced happiness, satisfaction, confidence, and inner strength.

2. Evoke the feelings and stay with them for a while, then answer this question: How do you feel about yourself as a result of doing this?

3 Doing this helps you realize that you can evoke and keep alive good, healthy feelings at will.

4. Gaining the power of positive feelings and the ability to use this power constructively depends on you doing this for yourself—without falling back on old habits.

Our Body Is Our Castle

Our body is our home in which Spirit lives and breathes. When it fails to get nurturing attention, it seeks attention from injurious sources and its well--being suffers. The purer the care our body receives—especially care that is non-judgmental and compassionate—the more it thrives. We can care for our body through gentle massages, touching, grooming, and more. These relaxing actions restore health and improve our well-being while they nurture our souls.

Once you truly accept your new image and fall in love with it, you will be able to tap into your Inner World. Once you understand and accept your Inner World, it's easy to do the same for your Outer World! Today, here are the messages I would like to convey to you.

1. Keep your head up high! Don't feel ashamed of anything. You know you didn't commit a crime by getting sick. Your illness wasn't a punishment for past transgression. Focus on what you have yet to learn from it.

2. Feel that you are a desirable woman, even with one breast. Change your outlook on life, realizing that other virtues are more important to your existence including forgiveness, compassion, a positive attitude and a good sense of humor.

In Eastern culture, there is no separation between the body and the spirit. As the saying goes, "Healthy Spirit in a Healthy Body." I share the following exercises that may help you regain health in both your spirit and body.

A Gem Needs Polishing to Shine

Humans will always encounter crises. Since the beginning of time, we've been called upon to deal with them. Close scrutiny shows us that most crises are opportunities for growth. Through them, we can either advance or stay where we are. We can experience either inspiration or desperation.

Personal growth is the process of responding positively to change. Whatever comes our way, we can give it meaning and transform it into something of value. Like a precious gem, it can't be polished without friction, nor can humanity be perfected without trials and tribulations. Today, you can choose to turn obstacles into strengths by being a model of inspiration to yourself and for other women in your situation—to shine and reshape attitudes into precious gems.

When you feel down, begin the habit of asking questions of your intuition.

"What is it that I am here to understand?"

"What is the best possible outcome for this situation?"

"What kind of life lesson am I to learn from this situation?"

The answers will not always leap into your mind. It takes time to train yourself to "hear" the subtle messages from your inner guidance. Often, the answers come as a quiet impulse to try something different, or a gradual awakening to a new way of dealing with an obstacle. Work diligently to remind yourself that your intuition could help guide you to peace of mind in any situation.

Eventually, you will find the answers that will help you to overcome your fears of intimacy after mastectomy, and educate and enlighten the man in your life.

Consider your mastectomy ordeal as a wake-up call from a higher power.

You are not a victim, and God is not punishing you for any transgression!

Meditation and Happiness

Meditation relaxes the body and mind and eases tension, evoking feelings of peacefulness and bliss. While meditating, allow few thoughts to pass through your mind. For a while, these thoughts lose their power. You'll experience peace of mind, which allows happiness to show itself.

Meditation Exercise

1. Sit down comfortably in a quiet place. Hold your back straight. Relax your body and breathe a few slow, deep breaths. Concentrate on your awareness, on your being. Penetrate into your inner "I."

2. Concentrate on the feeling of awareness and being alive. Don't pay attention to any single thought. When you get distracted by your thoughts, imagine them floating by on a cloud.

3. Continue contemplating without fighting with your thoughts or tensing your body.

4. Take it easy. Regard your meditation as a pleasant game. Keep focusing on the being you know you are. Focus on the quality of your thoughts, on your inner being.

---

5. Let yourself sink into this meditation without any tension for 10 minutes. Just stay with the feeling of calmness that you experience.

6. Let this feeling grow and you'll begin to know what peace of mind and happiness are. Meditating may be difficult at first, so be gentle with yourself as you learn this new skill. If you persevere day after day, you will learn.

While happiness comes from the inside, waiting to be discovered, thoughts, desires, and habits sometimes hide your true happiness. You become restless. One way to access that positive feeling is in meditation. Let your mind become calm again to allow the depths of happiness to surface.

When you meditate, the quieter your mind is, the more peace of mind you possess and the more happiness you experience. Calm your mind through meditation and you will be happy and be able to handle obstacles much more easily.

Over time and with more practice, it becomes easier to silence the chatter that naturally occurs in your mind when you are still. Hear the happiness you were born to experience. The more you meditate, the more this state will regenerate itself and show up in your daily life as well.

Experiencing and repeating meditation will make you an expert at tuning into your inner spirit and finding peace of mind.

Befriend Your Body

Our body is an amazing complex mechanism that serves us throughout our entire lives. It takes care of us even when we are asleep. The body has a certain wisdom of its own. Thank your body. Be grateful for it. Listen to it. Go for walks, rest, breathe, do things that your body enjoys doing out of sheer enjoyment of being alive. Do not fight with your body. It is not your foe, it is your friend. Treat it as such and show reverence for it. It is nature's gift to you.

Benefits of Meditation

By being in harmony with your body you will also be in harmony with nature, with existence. Instead of going against the current, go with the current. Allow life to happen. There is nothing more divine and valuable than life itself. Respect your body, cherish your body, and your body will respond accordingly.

The Healing Power of Solitude

Some of the greatest people of all time have practiced solitude regularly. They've learned how to use silence to still their minds and tap into their subconscious powers for answers to their questions.

You, too can get in touch with your own intuition and make decisions about your own life rather than responding to the pressures of what other people think you should do. It is necessary to break the hold of conventional wisdom and go within to the wisdom of the heart. You can do this through meditation or by simply seeking solitude and entering into a few moments of quiet reflection regularly. This activates the heart-mind connection and enables you to listen deeply. When all is still within, you will know you have contacted your heart-mind center.

Your feelings and your emotions are the access point to the inner powers of your mind. The most important part of getting in touch with your feelings is to practice solitude on a regular basis. Solitude is the most powerful activity in which you can engage. People who practice it correctly and frequently never fail to be amazed at the difference it makes in their lives.

Most people are so busy "being busy" and "doing something" it's highly unusual for them to deliberately sit and do nothing. As motivational speaker Brian Tracy said "People begin to become great when they begin to take time quietly by themselves, when they begin to practice solitude."

The incredible thing about solitude is that, when practiced correctly, it works close to 100% of the time. While you are sitting there, a river of ideas will flow through your mind. You'll think about countless subjects in an uncontrolled stream of consciousness. Thank goodness your job is just to relax and listen to your inner voice.

At a certain stage during your period of solitude, the answers to the most pressing difficulties facing you (for example, your health) will emerge quietly and clearly, like a boat putting in gently to the side of a lake.

These answers will come so clearly and feel so perfect that you'll experience a deep sense of gratitude and contentment.

When you emerge from this period of quiet, do exactly the actions that come to you. That could involve dealing with your health, starting something, quitting something. Whatever it is, when you follow the guidance you received in solitude, it will turn out to be exactly the right thing to do. In addition, it will usually work out far better than you could have imagined. Just try it and see.

As you develop the habit of listening to yourself and then acting on the guidance you receive, you'll trust yourself more and more.

You Are Priceless

At my seminars, I usually start my seminar by holding up a $50 bill in front of a room of 100 people. Then I ask, "Who would like to have this fifty-dollar bill?"

Hands start going up.

Then I say: "I am going to give this fifty-dollar bill to one of you, but first let me do this." I crumple it up and ask, "Who still wants it?"

Hands stayed up in the air.

Next, I drop the bill on the ground and start to grind it into the floor with my shoe. I pick up the crumpled and dirty bill.

"Now, who still wants it?"

Still their hands were up.

"My friends, we have all learned a very valuable lesson. No matter what was done to this bill, you still wanted it because it did not decrease in value. It was still worth $50."

"Many times in our lives, we are all dropped, crumpled, and ground into the dirt by circumstances. We feel as though we are worthless. Nevertheless, no matter what has happened or what will happen, we will never lose our value. Dirty or clean, crumpled or finely creased, with one breast or none, we are still priceless. Always remember that! And let us not allow anyone to think we are less than whole!"

In Appendix A, you can find all the suggestions, exercises and tools that will help you to achieve the state of mind you desire. These exercises will help you to connect with your core being. You will realize that you are not only your body and you are not just your breast.

Repeat the affirmations below every day. Really believe it, and feel the excitement of each one of them when you repeat it to yourself.

You will be pleasantly surprised how these affirmations will build your confidence to accept your new image and you will love it!

---

1. I am love.
2. I love myself—body, mind and soul.
3. A well of love resides within me.
4. True happiness resides within me.

CHAPTER 7

The Will to Survive

Balance and Harmony

My savior during this time was my spiritual training and the spiritual 'toolbox' on which I relied. Without them, I imagine I would have fallen apart completely. I realized my being was out of balance. My physical being was only one aspect of the four necessary elements of life: mental, emotional, spiritual, and physical.

It's amazing how these four elements co-mingle and depend on one another. With the absence or weakening of one, disharmony can appear in the form of disease or illness. And any degree of disharmony can change the whole picture.

To help you understand try this exercise:

---

1. Close your eyes and imagine standing on the center of a table that has four steady legs. You feel comfortable. You can even open your legs to two corners of the table and still feel in control, safely maintaining your balance.

> **2.** Close your eyes again and imagine yourself standing on the center of a table that has one broken or crooked leg. How do you feel now? Do you feel safe and steady? Do you feel out of balance? Do you fear that you'll fall?

Similarly, when one aspect of your life is in disharmony with the rest of the elements, you'll likely feel shaky and unstable, living in fear that you'll fall.

That's exactly where I was those days, standing on a table with broken legs trying to find balance. However, as soon as I was able to think more clearly, I knew I had to reevaluate my priorities. I needed to use my spiritual tools to help me realize that my quality of life didn't depend on living with one breast or even no breasts. *It depended on my attitude and perceptions of life.* Consequently, I had to make drastic changes.

The purpose of this exercise is for you to create a balance in your life by using the exercises that the Wise Man recommends.

What causes out-of-balance situations and illnesses? In one word—stress. Even Western medicine recognizes that stress plays a large role in most diseases.

Stress often results from how we've been raised, the values and beliefs we learned in childhood, and our overall attitude toward life. In contrast, happiness comes from our souls, from our mental, emotional, and spiritual states of mind. It comes from the core of our beings. It comes from the attitudes we embrace at every moment of our lives which, in turn, determine how we react to any incident we experience.

How do we find balance so we can live in harmony with all aspects of our lives?

For me, it was changing my belief systems and overall attitude toward daily living. That required channeling new energy that came from new beliefs and attitudes to the other elements in my life. After all, energy powers everything—every positive or negative thought, every daydream or deliberate visualization, any good or bad vibrations that get registered in our subconscious minds. Everything in the Universe is energy. We see differences because each object has a different wavelength and density.

We live in an ocean of energy, with each wave in this ocean influencing other waves. As part of this ocean of energy, thoughts interact with the creative Universal energy. Where energy gets channeled depends on choice.

After the removal of my infected implant, I chose to channel my energy toward helping people with situations similar to mine. My mission is to awaken their dormant senses, empower and inspire them to overcome obstacles in their lives, and find stability while standing at the center of that table.

Blessing in Disguise

At times, I have come to call my challenge with cancer a "blessing in disguise" because I caught it early enough, thanks to my spiritual awareness. If I hadn't, I doubt I'd be around today to tell my story. My outlook, my perspective toward life, and my priorities have all changed for the better. I enjoy living in a completely new way. My life is fuller and richer now. I appreciate every moment, consciously making decisions that correspond to how I want to feel in the moment. I make time to take a walk every morning, smell the roses, listen to the birds chirping, talk to my plants, and listen to the silence. Most of all, I feel precious life all around me.

Even though I cannot wear bikinis anymore, I love to go swimming in a one-piece bathing suit. If people stare at me, it doesn't bother me—I don't feel I am less of a woman because I have only one breast. Interestingly enough, in my first forty-five years, I had received only three marriage proposals, but since my breast cancer, I've received two. Go figure! I have my own theories about this phenomenon. Either the men feel sorry for me and want to make me feel better, or they think that I am a "desperate housewife" and would accept any proposal. Or maybe, just maybe, sexuality springs from self-acceptance and exudes from inside of us. We need to learn to love ourselves, falling in love with our new image. When we adopt these qualities, we automatically exude self-confidence and create a new aura around us. Before we know it we will turn ourselves into a magnet to attract men. And it has nothing to do with any part of our body, but has every thing to do with our personality and attitude.

It may sound like a cliché for me to call my cancer a blessing in disguise. However, many times I ask if my life would have been as rich as it is today if I hadn't traveled along this path. It's a journey that has been enriched by many courageous women. And I know the principles I've used along the way have worked for others like Pam Rehwald as well.

Never Failing Faith and Hope

I first met Pam on a conference call. We immediately liked each other and exchanged phone numbers so we could stay in touch. Because Pam was living in Seattle and I was in California, it was hard to meet face to face. But that didn't stop us from sharing our experiences about cancer. Luckily, within two months, we did meet at a seminar in Los Angeles. I was struck by this tall, elegantly dressed lady who wore a hat and a beautiful smile. I was amazed by her story.

Pam's battle with cancer started at age 17 when she had surgery to remove a benign lump in her breast. Twenty years later, she began having miserable headaches. She'd take aspirin and go right back to work until one Wednesday, she was so exhausted, she lay down to nap and didn't wake up until the following Sunday. When she did wake up, she didn't recognize her four children or her husband. She didn't know who or where she was. Something was obviously wrong.

After a myriad of doctors' visits and tests, Pam was diagnosed with a type of brain tumor known as astrocytoma. The doctors ruled it "inoperable" and gave her a 50-50 chance of surviving one year.

All energy drained, Pam and her husband wondered how something unexpected like this could happen to them. "We walked to the car crying. It was awful," she recalled. When they got home, Pam got on her knees and asked God to give her strength and hope to overcome this tragedy. She'd always had undeniable faith that she could go through a crisis and come out of it better than ever. And that's exactly what she set out to do.

At the time, Pam and her husband had a thriving artwork business. They had just bought a house and she thought their lives were moving forward smoothly. Suddenly, they had to give up their home, their business, and any possessions they couldn't afford anymore to cover medical expenses.

Pam chose to have radiation on her tumor. After being given a 50-50 odds to survive, what other options did she have? She underwent 6,000 rads of radiation therapy and started losing her hair—not a pleasant experience for any woman.

Yet she kept strong her faith that she could cure herself, so she put her energy into doing just that—healing. She started picking up rocks that were the same size as her tumor and put them in her bedside drawer. Every night, she reached into the drawer, picked up the rocks and held them, rubbing each one in her hand while she visualized her tumor shrinking.

She did this ritual for six weeks, all the time believing in her heart the tumor was getting smaller and smaller. One night, she stuck her hand into the drawer and couldn't find any of the rocks. She got so excited, she yelled to her husband, "My tumor is gone, my tumor is gone!" A few months later, she declared to her doctors that her tumor had disappeared. After about a year, they finally agreed with her; they could find no traces of it.

Ten years later, Pam started having seizures. The doctors diagnosed a second brain tumor of a rare type called an oligodendroglioma and gave her only a few months to live. "Go home and write your will," one doctor recommended. But Pam refused to give up. She went to see Dr. Mitchell Berger, a neurosurgeon.

Deeming it a terminal situation, Dr. Berger proposed a radical kind of surgery to remove the tumor on the left side in a complex part of Pam's brain that not only controlled her dominant hand but also her language functions. Once again, dying was not an option in her mind. "Hell, no! I'm not leaving this planet yet," she declared and chose to undergo the surgery.

Pam stayed awake under mild sedation during the nine-hour surgery. Dr. Berger removed most of her temporal lobe while sparing the islands of functional cortex responsible for her cognitive functions. She spent five days in the Intensive Care Unit, followed by a year of chemotherapy and subsequent years of gradual improvement.

The Comeback Kid

Yes, Pam did survive and, with all her faith and determination behind her, decided to excel! After her surgery, she had to learn to walk, talk, read, and write all over again like a six-year-old child even though she was in her late forties. In addition to losing a quarter of her brain, she lost her husband to divorce—he couldn't handle the stress of Pam's illness and recovery—and one of her sons left, too.

Despite her tragedies, Pam never gave up and she fully recovered. As she said:

Since my second brain tumor surgery, I always had a feeling someone was watching over me. I believe I survived by my strong faith, attitude, and sense of humor. That strength comes from feeling

a direct connection to God if one is willing
to go with it.

Currently, she's pursuing a career as an artist
and inspirational speaker. As she says, "Miracles do
happen. God put me back on Earth after two brain
tumors and two out-of-body experiences to tell my
story." Pam's business card describes her as "The
Comeback Kid" and her motto is: "Never, Ever Give
Up."

When Pam saw the doctor who had advised her
to write her will ten years earlier, he couldn't believe
his eyes. No, Pam did *not* write her will. Instead, she
used her will power to survive and to tell her story of
overcoming loss, pain, and hardship. Today, she enjoys
a positive and hope-filled life, using her sense of humor,
squeezing every drop of juice out of life that she can,
and never, ever giving up. To Pam, squeezing every
drop of juice out of life means to:

1. Live life to its fullest potential.
2. Open your heart and mind to a world
    where   all things are possible.
3. Pursue your dreams with everything
    that's within you.
4. Stretch yourself and go beyond the
    known into the unknown.
5. Follow your heart and fulfill the desires
    that inspire you.
6. Forgive others and find true freedom
    and peace of mind.
7. Take a leap of faith in the process of life,
    trusting everything will be all right.

8. Take control of what you can and accept what you can't.
9. Never give up on your dreams.
10. Focus on what's really important to you.
11. See others through the eyes of compassion.
12. Take action in spite of your fears.
13. Discover that fear is an illusion.
14. Feel the fear and do it anyway.
15. Say "I love you" more often.
16. Breathe deeply and let worries dissolve.
17. Understand that we don't own anything; we just get to use things for a while.

Pam's website is: http://www.hope-is-being-alive.com
Pam's email address is: faithpam@juno.com

"You must give some time to your fellow men. Even if it's a little thing, do something for others - something for which you get no pay but the privilege of doing it."
- Albert Schweitzer

CHAPTER 8

My Two Mothers

A family is a place where minds come in contact with one another. If these minds love one another the home will be as beautiful as a flower garden. But if these minds get out of harmony with one another it is like a storm that plays havoc with the garden." -Buddha

So much of my journey relates to two influential women I call my biological mother and my spiritual mother. I would like to share with you my experiences with them.

My Biological Mother

My biological mother, Hannah Yekutiel, grew up in Afghanistan practically without a mother. Her mother had passed away when my mother was very young. As a result, she didn't really have a childhood. In those days, people got married and had babies very young. My mother was fifteen years old when she gave birth to her first child. I'm the third child, after an older sister and brother. Four more babies followed me. Seven of us altogether grew up in Israel with the same parents and under the same roof.

Fortunately, when Israel became a state in 1948, 99% of the Jewish population in Afghanistan was able to fulfill their dreams and prayers of "next year in Jerusalem" when they moved to Israel. Like these Jews, my parents moved to Israel in 1953 when I was a few years old. During those years, people were moving there from all over the world and the country couldn't absorb all of them. Consequently, there was no housing, no jobs, and no food. It was a time of rationing, with the government giving coupons for essentials such as bread, butter, sugar, and eggs based on the number of people in a household. As children not knowing any differently, we were very happy. I remember eating a sandwich spread with margarine and brown sugar sprinkled on the top. To me, it was delicious. Everything we ate was delicious, like manna from heaven.

Being a good businessman as my father had been in Afghanistan didn't help him in Israel; however, he had managed to transfer goods to Israel. Selling them enabled him to purchase a house for his family.

In fact, our family seemed well-off compared to many other immigrant families. Growing up in Israel during the birth of a new nation was an exciting time filled with pride. I considered my childhood happy and healthy, even though I sensed the hardship my parents were going through. I loved school and was a good student eager to learn. I was popular among my classmates at elementary school. Upon turning 18 years old, I did my compulsory service in the Israeli army for one-and-a-half years it was a fun and rewarding time in my life.

While growing up, I never had anybody in my family to look up to or ask for advice or support. Even though I had two older siblings, I made all of my own decisions and became self reliant at a very young age. Because I was doing well in all aspects of my life, I became the center of my family. As it turned out, I virtually became my mother's mother. She'd often turn to me for advice about her problems. So did my siblings.

A New Motherland

In 1972 at the age of 27, I came to the United States to visit and ended up in Los Angeles where my oldest brother already was living. This visit was meant to last only three weeks but I loved the Los Angeles lifestyle and stayed for three months. I made many friends, went to school to improve my English, and had a marvelous time. I didn't want to go back to Israel. However, I had a job waiting for me there, so I returned with a plan to come back to Los Angeles permanently sometime in the future.

Two days before the Yom Kippur War broke out In October 1973, I left Israel for California and stayed with friends I'd met there on my first visit. They offered me a job as well. I lived with them for six weeks until I got my driver's license and purchased a car, and then found my own apartment.

For the first time in my life, I was totally on my own. I was in heaven! It felt as if I were on a vacation, without having anybody else's burden on my shoulders. I worked as an accountant while investing in real estate and other ventures. Curious to learn how people in the other part of our planet lived, I traveled quite a bit.

The Los Angeles economy in the early 90's wasn't vibrant or encouraging. In 1990, my life took a big turn when I lost all my assets, my entire life's savings. My younger brother and his family in L.A. moved back to Israel for good. He and my mother talked me into moving back, too, which I did in October 1993.

In Israel, I rented an apartment from one of my sisters and tried to build a new life. I struggled financially and promises of support from my mother didn't come through. It felt as though all my siblings were against me, too. How ironic! I was back in the country where I grew up and was surrounded by family members—a picture-perfect situation in the eyes of outside observers. So far as my family thought, what more could I ask for?

Home Without a Home

Still, nothing was going my way. I had a hard time finding a suitable job and worked as a secretary. Mostly, I couldn't handle being told I was "too old" to perform a number of jobs, even though I was only in my early fifties. Besides, I'd always felt self-reliant and earned money without asking for help. I'd often helped my siblings financially and emotionally. In this situation, I felt dependent on family members while being surrounded by some who resented me. I became a stranger in a strange land with no one in whom to confide. Added to that, I was so depressed I couldn't sleep at night or think clearly.

I realized I'd made a mistake moving back to Israel. *How could I be so gullible, naïve, vulnerable, and trusting to believe that the situation that I ran away from twenty years earlier had changed with my family?* In fact, now it was much worse. Every day, I wondered how I could get out of this situation which went on for almost three years.

One day, I went to get a gas mask from one of the government offices because Iraq's then President Saddam Hussein was threatening to use nuclear weapons on Israel. There, I saw people shoving and fighting to grab the gas masks as if there weren't enough for everyone. I walked away from the scene realizing that it wasn't Saddam Hussein who would kill me: it was the highly stressful negative environment in which I was living. *How could I have been so short-sighted, so blind to come back?*

At that moment, I decided to return to the States immediately. I bought a one-way ticket to Los Angeles, packed two suitcases, and left Israel on January 9, 1997, leaving behind my most treasured belongings. When I landed at LAX, I started making calls to find a place to stay temporarily. Thankfully, I received an invitation to stay at the home of my girlfriend Rivka Horowitz the same Ricki who later would faithfully taken care of me when I was to go through surgical treatment. I immediately started looking for a job. I ended up staying with dear Ricki for four months. Although I was eternally grateful for her kindness and hospitality, I wanted to have my own place and find peace of mind, so I rented an apartment and moved out.

A few months later, I flew back to Israel to sell my belongings and send the rest to L.A. I was shocked to find that most of my belongings were missing, broken, or destroyed. Apparently, my sister's son and his friend moved into the apartment and made it comfortable for themselves. They turned it into a bachelor pad with my sister's permission. They used some of my belongings that were useful to them and discarded the rest. They moved some of my furniture and other belongings to my sister's house. I packed whatever I could salvage of the few art objects still in good condition and shipped them to Los Angeles.

My sister wouldn't let me be in the apartment unless she was present. She wouldn't even let me in her house unless she herself was there. Her behavior made me feel utterly rejected and mortified me so much that I went into a state of shock, which led to severe hair loss a few weeks later. If only I realized then that the hair loss outwardly mirrored the deep loss of my possessions, fueled by my resentment of my sister.

I couldn't even tell my other sisters what had happened because I was so embarrassed. I could not comprehend how a sister could do such a thing. However, I told my mother briefly about what my sister did with my belongings. She wasn't surprised. She had even noticed different furniture in my sister's house and asked if it was new. My sister answered, "No. It's Lea's." Then my mother told me that what happened was my fault for trusting my sister after leaving everything behind. I was not surprised by my mother's reaction. I didn't expect her to do anything. My mother's influence over her children depended on if her own interests were served. Only then would she take sides. Otherwise, she'd ignore issues, especially at this ripe stage of her life.

Moreover, my sister had control over my mother's financial affairs and she was one of the two proclaimed to be her favorite children. Even though she'd given birth to seven of us, in her mind, she had only two favorites and I wasn't one of them.

I had no idea then that my mother's resentment of me directly seeded my lack of self-acceptance. It is well known in alternative healing that the left side of our body correlates with the feminine principle, while the right corresponds to the masculine principle. It was no mistake that my breast cancer manifested on the left side of my body. Perhaps the high value I placed on the crowning glory of my female physique—my breasts—harbored the paramount life lesson I needed to learn; namely that of embracing my own true feminine identity. I could interpret the surgical reconstruction of my left breast symbolic of the spiritual reconstruction that my feminine principle had to undergo.

Ultimately, the above incident with my family reminded me why I had originally left Israel—and why I returned to L.A. It was my heroine's journey to find another mother—one who would rebirth not my physical body, but my spiritual one.

My Spiritual Mother

The first time I met Virginia Downsbrough was in 1987 through a pilot seminar that was cut short due to an emergency. To make up for it, anyone who didn't finish the seminar was invited to complete it with Virginia at her center in Montecito, California.

Virginia was tall with pure snow white hair and piercing baby blue eyes, which gave her a distinguished and striking appearance. Even though she had a wrinkled face and body, she seemed ageless. She was in her seventies, I guessed, but her chronological age was insignificant because of the contagious energy she emanated.

I spent many weekends at Virginia's Montecito retreat home where I learned more about Virginia, who had devoted her life to self-growth and spiritual enlightenment. After moving from Los Angeles to Montecito, she created her self-growth business—a prospering one—called The Advanced Ability Center.

Her house on the top of Montecito Hills had breathtaking views from every angle. Its high windows faced the ocean and no drapes blocked the view. Two sides faced the ocean, allowing participants to see the sunrise and sunset, as well as an avocado orchard and mountain homes with beautiful architecture. Even when we were indoors, we felt immersed in the beauty of the outdoors.

Virginia had turned this place into an oasis by planting an array of flowers in rainbow colors with different shapes and textures around the house. Picture perfect! Spending time surrounded by this beauty and Virginia's personal touch made us feel closer to God. That's where I was years later on a retreat at her home when I had experienced the dark cloud hovering over me.

Virginia the Healer

I recall once when I was sick. I felt as if a needle was stuck in my throat. I couldn't swallow anything and was taking antibiotics that weren't helping. One Sunday morning, I couldn't stand the pain and so I called Virginia. She told me to drive up to see her. Despite the cold, pouring winter rain in Los Angeles, I was sweating profusely and was concerned about the weather. Virginia wouldn't hear any of my excuses. She kept repeating, "Get into your car and bring your body over here."

I drove through the torrential rain. When I arrived, I joined her students in several exercises about beliefs. The purpose of the exercises was to learn how to gain control over one's life instead of being at the effect of circumstances (like the pouring rain). After doing these exercises, I realized all the needle-like symptoms in my throat had disappeared. I never got sick again with the same symptoms. As I stated earlier, after coming back from Israel and being severely upset about my experience with my sister, my mind and body went into a prolonged state of shock. Before long, I was finding fallen hair everywhere: in the shower, in my bed, on the kitchen floor. I also noticed the hair gradually thinning at the front of my scalp.

Although I knew I was losing my hair due to stress from quarreling with my sister, I didn't know what to do about it except panic. I did go to a dermatologist who prescribed Rogaine, a liquid that's supposed to stop hair from thinning. I used it a few times and hated its side effects. My hair became coarse and turned a grayish color. The last time I used it, I got dizzy and almost passed out. Another doctor simply told me she didn't have any solution for my problem and suggested that I "just get used to it"—that is, accept that I was going bald. I refused to live with a "bad hair day" every day for the remainder of my life.

At that point, I had a moment of total clarity and realized I was concentrating on the fruits—the results—instead of the roots—the cause of the results. I had to handle this stress on an emotional and spiritual level instead of on a physical level. So I called Virginia and drove to Montecito to discuss with her my hair loss. She suggested doing this simple exercise on forgiving. It is called the Compassion Exercise. I closed my eyes, put my attention on the person I needed to forgive, and repeated these words to myself:

Compassion Exercise

- Just like me, this person is seeking happiness in her life.

- Just like me, this person has known sadness, loneliness, and despair.

- Just like me, this person is trying to avoid suffering in her life.
- Just like me, this person is learning about life.

While doing the exercise, put yourself in their situation and imagine feeling how they are feeling. In addition to that, repeat the following statements to yourself:

1. I now release all the negative energy that influenced my life and forgive those people who harmed me.

2. I choose to live in divine inspiration.

3. I am grateful for divine inspiration.

Release any negative energy and let it drain out into the Universe.

Slowly, I released my negative energy. I let it drain out of me and into the Universe. By doing this, I was able to forgive my sister completely. And of course, my hair loss stopped immediately. I knew that if I had kept holding grudges and refused to forgive, I would be completely bald by now.

Who knows what other physical symptoms this kind of negativity would have created in my life?

An Exercise of Forgiveness

"Forgiveness is the key that unlocks the door of resentment and the handcuffs of hate. It is a power that breaks the chains of bitterness and the shackles of selfishness." — William Arthur Ward

Here is a short exercise that can help you unlock the door of resentments and release the pain you feel. Ask yourself these five questions:

Forgiveness Exercise

1. Against whom am I holding a grudge right now, today, at this moment? List as many as necessary.

2. In what way does holding these grudges enhance my life and bring me peace?

3. In what way does holding these grudges restrict me? (e.g., limits my joy and happiness, health, relation

---

ships, career, finances, self-esteem,
stress, etc.)

4.   Am I going to continue paying these
      prices and placing my attention on
      what I do NOT want more of in my
      life?

5.   Alternatively, do I choose to MAKE
      PEACE? Make a note to yourself:
      How did you feel after you released
      the negative energy and forgave
      yourself and others?

      Use this exercise to forgive yourself
      and other people in your life.
      Remember, as long as you hold
      grudges against anyone who has
      harmed you, you give that person
      control over your life.

Having Virginia to turn to for advice and spiritual
guidance felt so good, especially since I never had
family members or teachers who I could ask for help.
Virginia filled that gap when I was in my fifties. She
made me feel warm and fuzzy inside and not alone.
Virginia came to be the mother figure—the image of a
true mother that I'd hoped for and expected of my
biological mother. During this time, she accepted me
unconditionally and was always there for me and for
many others.

Between surgeries, I found a sanctuary from the
doctors when I called Virginia and spent a few days in

her tranquilizing presence and surroundings. During the years that I knew her, we developed such an unusual friendship, trust and intimacy that I felt comfortable turning to her with any issues in my life. It was a new experience for me and I treasured it. There were always students staying at her house to take the Avatar course she taught. Even though this course was being taught all over the world, people would come from thirty-five states and twenty-five countries to take the course with Virginia. She touched many people's lives.

She would do exercises with her students and help them to overcome hurdles in their lives. The whole environment played a critical role on my own healing journey. I am extremely grateful to have had Virginia my spiritual mother, the tower of strength during my ordeal with cancer.

The following are some of the simple yet powerful exercises she taught:

Gratitude Exercise

Concentrate on different objects and notice little details about them. Move from one object to the next and count them all. These exercises draw attention away from the body and quiet the mind.

While doing them, I would also state things for which I was grateful, such as:

1.   I am grateful I am still alive.

---

2. I am grateful I detected my cancer in the early stages, thanks to my spiritual awareness.

3. I am grateful for having only one breast affected with cancer instead two.

4. I am grateful the cancer didn't spread to any other part of my body.

5. I am grateful I had the ability to forgive myself and forgive others.

6. I am grateful I didn't have to go through chemotherapy or radiation.

Virginia Leaves the Earth

At age 86, Virginia herself was diagnosed with cancer. She had been a heavy smoker and even though she'd stopped smoking years earlier, its destruction had caught up with her. For one whole year, she fought the illness with every ounce of energy she had in her. She went though repeated surgeries and blood transfusions, which was dangerous at her advanced age. I stayed in touch with her family during all this time. She had so many near-death experiences, they had stopped counting.

Just a few months later, she would be diagnosed with another type of cancer. But this time, she didn't have the energy to fight it. Within twelve hours of entering hospice care, she passed away, surrounded by her family.

Her passing devastated me. I'd lost my mentor and spiritual mother who had helped me to mold my life as an adult. She'd become my dear and intimate friend.

Wherever you are, Virginia, know that I am thinking of you!

"The best thing to give to your enemy is forgiveness; to an opponent, tolerance; to a friend, your heart!"
- Benjamin Franklin

CHAPTER 9

Spiritual Beings Having a Human Experience

"You are not in the body, the body is in you! The mind is in you! They happen to you. They are there because you find them interesting."
— Sri Nisargadatta Maharaj

All illness stems from a state of dis-ease and stress that affects our psyche and eventually manifests in our bodies as illness. When I was struggling most with cancer, I realized that Western medicine wasn't capable of dealing with a person as a whole being. I needed to look for alternative healing for my broken spirit. As the great philosopher Pierre Teilhard de Chardin said: "We are not human beings having a spiritual experience. We are spiritual beings having a human experience."

I've had always kept an open mind about alternative healing techniques, finding myself drawn to Eastern healing and its ancient wisdom. In addition, weSPARK made several therapies available through classes such as yoga, Qi-Gong, Tai-Chi, and integrative energy work. I believe we are spiritual beings having a human experience on Earth.

Nurturing Your Body

Your body is an entity that loves you unconditionally. It does whatever you want and never questions you. When you start communicating with your body, talk with your body and ask what it wants. When you love yourself and your new image, you are happy and it reflects on your surrounding. If you don't love yourself, it reflects on everything in your life. Allow everything to come to your life effortlessly.

This exercise will help you concentrate, calm your mind, open the energy centers of your body, and allow the natural healing life force to flow into every organ.

Nurturing Exercise

1. In private, secure and comfortable surroundings, remove your clothing and spend 10–15 minutes focusing attention on your body.

2. Apply soothing, aromatic lotion of your choice. Gently pat your body. Stroke it. Talk to it and admire it. Your purpose is to cherish what you have.

3. Affirm that you are accepting, forgiving, and loving.

4. Accept anything, considering anything with a defect or imperfection with the same compassion and understanding you would give to your best friend.

5. Consistently accept your new image lovingly, admiringly.

> 6.   Be patient with yourself as you do so.

The Power of Solitude

To get the full benefit of your periods of solitude, sit quietly for at least 30 to 60 minutes at a time. If you have not done this exercise before, it will take the first 25 minutes or so to stop fidgeting. Do not be surprised if you will have an almost irresistible desire to get up and do something. Persevere. Why? Because solitude

---

Solitude Exercise

1.   Relax completely. Breathe deeply. Let your mind flow. Don't deliberately think about anything.

2.   After 20 or 25 minutes, you'll begin to feel deeply relaxed and experience a flow of energy coming into your mind and body.

3.   You will have a tremendous sense of well-being. At this point, you'll be ready to get the full benefit of these moments of contemplation.

---

requires that you sit quietly, perfectly still, back and head erect, eyes open, without cigarettes, candy, writing materials, music, or any interruptions for at least 30 minutes or longer.

Ancient Chinese Healing Acupuncture

During my quest for spiritual and alternative healing, I came across the practice of acupuncture, the world's oldest method of healing spanning 3,000 years. Acupuncture uses fine needles made of metal, usually stainless steel. These needles are inserted through the skin into numerous points on the body. Based on Traditional Chinese Medicine, any disease or condition caused by an imbalance of energy in the body can be adjusted using acupuncture treatment, which brings a flood of energy flow to create a normal condition.

The body's energies circle through particular paths called meridians, which are like rivers flowing through the body to transport the energy (Chi or Qi in Chinese). That energy irrigates and nourishes tissues throughout the body. An obstruction in the movement of this river of chi imitates a dam in a stream—that is, it serves to back up the flow in one part of the body and restrict it in others.

I frequently use acupuncture treatments to relieve the pain in my left chest. Acupuncture helps to open up the channels of energy in my body, helping to distribute it through the rest of my body. These treatments took away the pain and helped me relax my body as well as my mind. Because acupuncture does not just treat the physical pain, it also helps to quiet the mind. I actually developed a great friendship with my acupuncturist. The relationship is warm and fuzzy and constitutes a kind of intimate caring. She always takes my pulse, checks my tongue and asks me if I am getting enough sleep. She cares about my well-being as a whole person and not just on a physical basis.

Acupuncture is a non-invasive treatment and has none of the side effects that Western medications introduce. I usually come out of my acupuncture treatments smiling, rejuvenated and relaxed—the pain in my chest vanished. It feels as if I had spent few hours at a luxurious spa.

Body, Mind, Spirit Activities

It has been said that there is nothing the wise man does reluctantly. I suggest that by doing these activities with great desire and intention, you'll find great healing.

1. Allow yourself time in each day to dream, desire, imagine, visualize yourself being healthy, cancer-free. Take time to flow energy and positive vibration in your body.

2. Every time you catch yourself with a negative train of thought, flip the switch to a warm, comfortable, positive feeling.

3. Whenever you feel down about yourself, stop. Regain your balance, and laugh out loud about it. Decide to consciously change the way you feel and make things better. Every "Feel Better" exercise will raise your positive vibration.

4. Every day, make a list of what you can laugh about, what brings you joy. Get excited over things big or small, and direct energy toward

them. Feel how it feels to have a healthy body and mind.

5. Constantly ask, "How am I flowing my energy? How am I flowing my energy? How am I flowing my energy?"

6. Write outrageously positive new scripts about your health every day.

7. Focus only on what you *intend* to have, instead of what you *don't* have.

8. Find new ways to feel better every day. Be creative. Be inventive. Be outrageous.

9. Accept for a final time that you are the *only* creator of your feelings.

10. Replace your "things to do" with a "things to feel" list. For example, go out and smell the roses. Determine how doing that makes you feel.

11. Keep your mind out of the past; it does not exist.

12. Start your day looking for positive aspects about your health, then deliberately seek them out and experience them. Start with being grateful for being alive. Be grateful to be able to smell the aroma of coffee or listen to the birds singing.

13. Stay alert to how you're feeling and the rest will be easy.

14. Pat yourself on the back for every perceived obstacle you created and turn it into opportunity.

15. Live in the *feeling place of your want* every day. You have dreams that have to be fulfilled. You have special places that you want to go and visit. Feel those dreams and feel those places in the present time—as if you are there right at the moment. Feel them the way you like them to be.

16. Speak tenderly to yourself *aloud* and feel how it feels.

17. Aim to feel good every day and watch how quickly what you want appears in your life.

18. Allow time to your health, overlooking thoughts about what you want *not* happening yet. It's on its way. Believe! Believe!

19. Believe in your own power. If you wake up feeling great, pump it. If you wake up feeling lousy, change it.

20. If something is bugging you, shift your thinking to a positive thought.

21. Listen to your guidance, and then act. Never, never, never act before you hear what "it" has to say.

22. Practice flowing appreciation into everything that crosses your path: a flower, a building, a lamp post in the street, a car that you like, people and animals.

23. Be thankful for every minute you live on planet Earth.

24. Calm down, relax, soften up, get natural, and get closer to *you*.

25. If all else fails, smile a phony smile. Just putting a smile on your face raises your vibrations.

26. Live in the present. That is why it's called a "present."

27. Know your body; you are the best doctor for yourself.

28. Listen to music that brings you joy.

29. Remember that nothing—*nothing*—is more important than feeling good, even if it is just feeling better. Open your heart to positive vibrations. Feelings are positive vibrations that bring joy and happiness.

30. Allow full health to come into your life. You deserve it!

"*Keep your Light shining, and let nothing deter you as you are more powerful than you realize, and nothing can move you from your path unless you allow it.*"
- Atmos through Mike Quinsey

Afterword

I have shared with you the darkest moments in my life. It has not been easy recalling unpleasant events I would rather forget. I have shed painful tears while reliving this mastectomy journey. Accepting the fact that I have to live with one breast for the remainder of my life has not been easy but, I did it and so can you! Forgiving the doctors who treated me has not been easy, but I did it to keep my own sanity. I am grateful for having you, the reader, to share my experiences. Writing this book helped me to heal the wounds.

You may or may not agree with everything I have attempted to convey here. You may or may not use the suggestions or exercises I've offered. If I've succeeded in opening your mind or getting you to consider another way of looking at your life, I have done my job. If anything I have shared here helps you to be gentler with yourself or helps you forgive yourself and others, I have done my job well.

And if you receive nothing else from this book, I hope you realize how unique you really are. Never give up on following your heart and accepting yourself as a whole woman!

Regardless of what you think of yourself
Regardless of what you think others think of you
Regardless of your perceived failures in life,
because you have one breast
Regardless of whoever you are with one breast or none
Regardless of wherever you are

Regardless of whatever you are doing in your life
Regardless of whoever you are with know that you are loved, you are valued, you are treasured and you are cherished by me.
Just because you are YOU.
Just because you are perfect exactly as you were born.
Just because you live and breathe.
Just because you are a light in the world.

I hope that by reading this book, it helped you to love, to value, to treasure and cherish yourself and believe that you deserve the best.

With much health, joy, love and laughter,

Lea Yekutiel

Please send your insights from reading this book to lea@ilovemybreastcancer.com. I'd love to receive your feedback.

For information on workshops and ezine subscription, visit my website:
http://www.ilovemybreastcancer.com

Appendix A

The following exercises were noted throughout this book. They are compiled here for easy reference, with additional exercises included. Enjoy!

Compassion Exercise

1. Close your eyes and put your attention on the person you need to forgive. Then repeat these words to yourself:

   Just like me, this person is seeking happiness in his/her life.
   Just like me, this person has known sadness, loneliness and despair.
   Just like me, this person is trying to avoid suffering in his/her life.
   Just like me, this person is learning about life.

   While doing the exercise, put yourself in the other person's situation and imagine feeling how he or she was feeling.

2. In addition, repeat the following statement to yourself:

   I now release all the negative energy that influenced my life and forgive those people who harmed me. I choose to live in divine inspiration. I am grateful for divine inspiration.

Slowly, release this negative energy.
Let it drain out of you and into the
Universe.

Forgiveness Exercise

William Arthur Ward wrote, *"Forgiveness is the
key that unlocks the door of resentment and the
handcuffs of hate. It is a power that breaks the chains
of bitterness and the shackles of selfishness."*

Here is a short exercise that can help you unlock
the door of resentments and release the pain you feel.
Ask yourself these questions:

1. Against whom am I holding a grudge
   right now, today, at this moment? List as
   many as necessary.

2. In what way does holding these grudges
   enhance my life and bring me peace?

3. In what way does holding these grudges
   restrict me? (e.g., limits my joy and
   happiness, health, relationships, career,
   finances, self-esteem, stress, etc.)

4. Am I going to continue paying these
   prices and placing my attention on what
   I do NOT want more of in my life?

5. Alternatively, do I choose to MAKE
   PEACE?

Make a note to yourself: How did you feel after you released the negative energy and forgave yourself and others? Use this exercise to forgive yourself and other people in your life. Remember, as long as you hold grudges against anyone who has harmed you, you give that person control over your life.

Simple Concentration Exercises

Gratitude Exercise

Concentrate on different objects and notice little details about them. Move from one object to the next and count them all. These exercises draw attention away from the body and quiet the mind. While doing them, also state things for which you are grateful.

- I am grateful for_____.
- I am grateful for_____.
- I am grateful for_____.
- I am grateful for_____.
- I am grateful for_____.
- I am grateful for_____.
- I am grateful for_____.

Nurturing Exercise

The purpose of this exercise is to help you concentrate, calm your mind, open the energy centers of your body, and allow the natural healing life force to flow into every organ.

1. In private, secure, and comfortable surroundings, remove your restricting clothing and spend 10 -15 minutes focusing attention on your body. Apply soothing, aromatic lotion of your choice.

2. Gently pat your body. Stroke it, talk to it, and admire it. Your purpose is to cherish what you have.

3. Affirm that you are accepting, forgiving, and loving.

4. Accept anything, considering anything with a defect or imperfection with the same compassion and understanding you would give to your best friend.

5. Consistently accept your new image lovingly, admiringly.

6. Be patient with yourself as you do so.

Meditation Exercise

1. Sit down comfortably in a quiet place, holding your back straight. Relax your body and breathe a few deep, slow breaths. Concentrate on your awareness, on your being. Penetrate into your inner "I."

2.   Concentrate on the feeling of awareness
      and being alive that you experience.
      Don't pay attention to any single thought.
      When you get distracted by your thoughts,
      imagine them floating by on a cloud.

3.   Continue contemplating without fighting
      with your thoughts or tensing your body.

4.   Take it easy. Regard your meditation as a
      pleasant game. Just keep focusing without
      words on the being you think you are.
      Don't focus on your body; focus on the
      quality of your thoughts, on your inner
      being.

5.   Let yourself sink into this meditation
      without any tension. Do this for 10 minutes
      and then just stay with the feeling of
      calmness that youexperience.

6.   Let this feeling grow and you'll begin to
      know what peace of mind and happiness
      are. Meditating may be difficult at first, so
      be gentle with yourself as you learn this
      new skill. If you persevere day after day,
      you will learn. Experiencing and repeating
      meditation will make you an expert at
      tuning into your inner spirit and finding
      peace of mind.

Solitude Exercise

To enjoy the full benefit of your periods of solitude, sit quietly for at least 30 to 60 minutes at a time. If you have not done this exercise before, it will take the first 25 minutes or so to stop fidgeting. You will almost have to hold yourself physically in your seat.

Do not be surprised if you will have an almost irresistible desire to get up and do something. You must persist. Why? Because solitude requires that you sit quietly, perfectly still, back and head erect, eyes open, without cigarettes, candy, writing materials, music, or any interruptions for at least 30 minutes or longer.

Become completely relaxed, breathe deeply. Let your mind flow. Don't deliberately think about anything. After 20 or 25 minutes, you'll begin to feel deeply relaxed and experience a flow of energy coming into your mind and body. You will have a tremendous sense of well-being. At this point, you'll be ready to get the full benefit of these moments of contemplation.

Body, Mind, Spirit Activities

It has been said that there is nothing the wise man does reluctantly. I suggest that by doing these activities with great desire, you'll find great healing.

1. Allow yourself time in each day to dream, desire, imagine, visualize yourself being healthy, cancer-free. Take time to flow energy and positive vibration in your body.

2. Every time you catch yourself with a negative train of thought, flip the switch to a warm, fuzzy, positive feeling.

3. Whenever you feel down about yourself, stop. Regain your balance, and laugh out loud about it. Decide to   consciously change the way you feel and make things better. Every "Feel Better" exercise will raise your positive vibration.

4. Every day, make a list of what you can laugh about, what brings you joy. Get excited over things big or small, and flow energy towards them. Sense how it feels to have a healthy body and mind.

5. Constantly ask, "How am I flowing my energy? How am I flowing my energy? How am I flowing my energy?"

6. Write outrageously positive new scripts about your health every day.

7. Focus only on what you *intend* to have, instead of what you *don't* have.

8. Find new ways to feel better every day. Be creative. Be inventive. Be outrageous.

9. Accept for a final time that you are the *only* creator of your feelings.

10. Replace your "things to do" with a "things to feel" list. For example, go out and smell the roses. Determine how doing that makes you feel.

11. Keep your mind out of the past; it does not exist.

12. Start your day looking for positive aspects about your health, then deliberately seek them out and experience them. Start with being grateful for being alive. Being grateful to be able to smell the aroma of coffee or listen to the birds singing.

13. Stay alert to how you're feeling and the rest will be easy.

14. Pat yourself on the back for every perceived obstacle you created and turn it into opportunity.

15. Live in the *feeling place of your want* every day. You have dreams that have to be fulfilled. You have special places that you want to go and visit. Feel those dreams and feel those places in the present time as if you are there right at the moment. Feel them the way you like them to be.

16. Speak tenderly to yourself *aloud* and feel how it feels.

17. Aim to feel good every day and watch how quickly what you want appears in your life.

18. Give time to your health, overlooking thoughts about what you want *not* happening yet. It's on its way. Believe! Believe!

19. Believe in your own power. If you wake up feeling great, pump it. If you wake up feeling lousy, change it.

20. If something is bugging you, shift your thinking to a positive thought.

21. Listen to your guidance, and then act. Never, never, never act before you hear what "it" has to say.

22. Practice flowing appreciation into everything that crosses your path: a flower, a building, a lamppost in the street, a car that you like, people and animals.

23. Be thankful for every minute you live on planet Earth.

24. Calm down, relax, soften up, get natural, and get closer to *you*.

25. If all else fails, smile a phony smile. Just putting a smile on your face raises your vibration.

26. Live in the present. That is why it's called a "present."

27. Know your body; you are the best doctor for yourself.

28. Listen to music that brings you joy.

29. Remember that nothing—*nothing*—is more important than feeling good, even if it is just feeling better. Open your heart to positive vibrations. Feelings are positive vibrations that bring joy and happiness.

30. Allow full health to come into your life. You *deserve* it!

Ten Simple Ways to Honor Your Uniqueness

"Everyone has his own specific vocation or mission in life; everyone must carry out a concrete assignment that demands fulfillment. Therein he cannot be replaced, nor can his life be repeated, thus, everyone's task is unique as his specific opportunity to implement it."
— Viktor Frankl

One message we hear from the time we are children is that it is better to give than receive. It is best to be humble. It is best to not shine a light on our selves.

True, and not so true! We also need to recognize that until we honor ourselves with love and compassion we will not be able to give fully to another or shine the light on another, nor will we truly understand humility.

These simple steps will take you on a path to honoring your uniqueness every day. Use them as a way to see how you are doing. Celebrate what is working, and choose to make adjustments where there is adjustment necessary.

1.   Take time for quiet daily. Yes, there is much that needs to get done. Once you maintain a habit of being quiet either to contemplate, pray, or meditate, you will be amazed how much more efficiently you will perform your tasks, duties and projects.

2. Treat yourself with as much care, if not more, than you treat others. Love and nurture yourself as you love and nurture those around you OR as you would LIKE to nurture those around you. Once you master caring for yourself, caring for others will become effortless and spring from the heart instead of from duty.

3. Graciously accept compliments from others. Never, ever disrespect the person you are complimenting by disregarding or negating their compliment. Instead, accept it as you would a treasure box or a long awaited gift. Be grateful they can see something extra special about you!

4. Spend time investing in and cultivating close friendships. Involve friends when building activities into your daily routine. Exercise with a friend, share meals together, keep in touch with a brief email or 10-minute daily phone call (time the call and keep the appointment.)

5. Surround yourself with beauty. Honor your home by decorating as a way to express who you are at your core. If you are bold, use bold colors and accessories. Light scented candles, listen to music you love, use soaps that are lathery and smell great. Go for the multi-sensory approach.

6.   Give joyfully and receive with open arms. Recognize that giving and receiving are on the same continuum and not separate at all! Learning to give completely translates into receiving more than you could ever plan or expect to receive. The results take care of themselves.

7.   Become a part of a larger community. This may mean a mastermind group or it may be a circle of friends or a book discussion group. Connect yourself with people who share your interests, goals and vision for the world. Synergy will empower you incredibly when you join in a community where you can equally give and receive on a very regular basis.

8.   Mentor someone simply for the pleasure of observing and becoming involved in their growth. Invite along for the ride with you someone who does not have the same education level or skills as you do. Listen to their input and see what you can create together. Chances are you will learn a lot from them (and vice versa!) creating a Win/Win situation as well as learning about your own strengths and weaknesses in the process.

9.   Live a purposeful, cause-oriented life. Recognize and embrace that you are creating your life as a masterful artist each

and every day. You can choose each day whether you want to simply let life happen each day or if you want to create it fully. Choose the latter.

10. Love yourself with all your heart, soul, and strength without attachment to what you are achieving in your life today. Be compassionate and understanding while also standing firm in the knowledge that you are both incredibly unique and incredibly capable.

When you can master this balance, being attached to your outcomes is not an issue because you will be achieving outcomes beyond your own imagination. You will be so magnetic, you will wonder where YOU have been all this time! The answer? You are RIGHT there, ready and waiting to follow these simple principles.

- Live with Passion. Today.
- You are special—don't ever forget it.
- Count your blessings, not your problems.
- Never be afraid to try something new.

And remember—amateurs built the ark; professionals built the Titanic.

Living in the Moment

"Realize deeply that the present moment is all you ever have."
—Eckhart Tolle

During my journey through enlightenment and spiritual growth, I noticed that most of the time when I was stressed out, worried, or unhappy, I was in the past or the future, which means "not in the moment." I also noticed that if I brought my attention back to the present, the pain, the stress, the worry, and the unhappiness disappeared almost immediately. This "living in the moment" idea may not be new to you since it has been discussed in the "spiritual" literature for many years.

What I am suggesting, however, is different from most literature in one very important way. Instead of the "idea" of living in the moment, I want you to "act on" living in the moment! That what's so exciting about it! You simply move your attention from the past to an environment where you passionately live in the present without an attachment to specific results. You will do what you do because you want to, not because you are afraid the past will repeat itself. Every moment you live is a "new unit of time." As soon as you understand the concept "new unit of time," you will always remember to live in the moment. *"He that never changes his opinions, never corrects his mistakes, will never be wiser on the to morrow than he is today."* —Tryon Edwards

The transition process may be tough at the beginning, but you are tougher! With practice and belief in yourself, it will become second nature.

Some years ago, I lived for six months in Montecito, California, at my spiritual master's home. She had a dog named Sugar. Sugar was very friendly and playful. She would come to my car to greet me when I came home. In the mornings, I would find her stretched out right next to my bed. Basically, we had a great relationship. Sugar was a member of the family. We even threw a birthday party for her with cake and birthday hats!

When circumstances brought me back to L.A., I didn't get the chance to visit Sugar for a while. A couple of months passed by before I could drive up to Montecito again. I was extremely disappointed when Sugar didn't greet me when I arrived. She didn't show any signs of recognition, totally ignoring me like I didn't exist in her world. Sugar's behavior did not make sense to me. All kind of thoughts were going through my head. *Is it possible that she totally forgot me? Are dogs susceptible to Alzheimer's disease like human beings?*

I was crushed. My feelings were hurt.

Then, all of a sudden, a light bulb went through my head. I looked at her and realized that she was "living in the moment." The past did not exist for her!

Wow! What a revelation! Sugar lives in the moment! What a wonderful way to live! Living in the moment is the ultimate way to live.

I felt a twinge in my heart. I actually was jealous of her ability to live in the moment. For just a little while, I wanted to be a dog in order to have that capability!

But if Sugar could live in the moment, why couldn't I live the same way?

A serious dialogue went on between my conscious mind and my subconscious mind. And then a brilliant idea crossed my mind. *If a dog can live in the moment, why can't I, too, live in the moment as a human being?*

At that "aha" moment, I changed my state of mind and adopted the notion of "living in the moment."

I love living in the moment! It doesn't mean that the past ceases to exist. The past does exist, but I don't let it to control my life in the NOW.

Attention and Focus

"All that we are is the result of what we have thought."
—**Buddha**

Few people realize the importance of directing and controlling our attention. The ability to be in present time with free-flowing attention, while deliberately directing that attention is the key to success in our lives.

Here are some questions you can ask yourself to find out how well you are able to control and direct your attention:

1. Do you compare yourself to others? Do you compare things in life to how you think they *should be* rather than enjoy how they *are*?

2. Do you think compassionate, caring thoughts about yourself or are your self-thoughts critical, harsh, or self-defeating?

3. Are you constantly wondering how others think about you and do you make decisions for yourself based on how you will look to others?

4. Do situations, issues, or events occur in your life that stick in your mind for hours, days, weeks, or even years?

5. Do you lack inner peace (or freedom from pain or anger) about these situations?

6. Is your mind quiet, or is there a lot of mind chatter?

7. Do you often get lost in daydreams or fantasies and then wonder why things don't get done or why your goals aren't achieved or why your life isn't the way you would like it to be?

8. Do you easily get distracted from a task, or a project or goal?

9. Is your mind clear most of the time or do you have a lot of mind fog and confusion?

10. Do you get discouraged and give up on a goal or a dream instead of being able to keep yourself going until you succeed?

11. Do you have goals and dreams but never let yourself really go for what you truly want because when you thin about them, one or more of these statements are true?

12. Do you have doubts and thoughts about them being too difficult to achieve?

13. Do you believe they will take too long?

14. Do you believe that you are too old now?

15. Do you believe they would take too much money?

16. Do you believe things like that happen for other people but not for you?

17. Do you believe you failed in the past, you will fail again—so why try?

18. What was your conclusion when doing the exercise above?

19. Were you thinking positively or negatively?

20. Do you believe you can succeed or are you trapped with negative self-talk that continues to keep you from getting all you deserve?

If you identified with these statements, even just a few, the way to break into the abundance that is waiting for you is to change your beliefs!

Appendix B

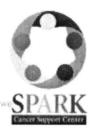

weSPARK Mission

weSpark is a special place dedicated to enhance the quality of life for cancer patients and their families and friends. weSPARK provides, free of charge, a center where one can join with others to share their experience, strength, and hope. weSpark offers multiple services designed to heal the mind, body and spirit of all those whose lives have been affected by cancer

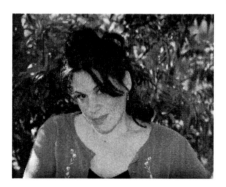

weSPARK Founder

Wendi Jo Sperber was an actress, mother and breast cancer warrior. When she was diagnosed in 1997, she was devastated, yet determined to live. She soon realized that although the physical treatment was difficult, the hardest battle was to be fought on the emotional front.

Wendie's dream was to open an independently-run cancer support center in a home-like setting.

In the fall of 2001 she opened weSPARK and her dream came true. weSPARK is a special place dedicated to enhancing the quality of life for cancer patients and their families and friends.

weSPARK provides a variety of programs and opportunities for social exchange to all people, regardless of income, race, religious affiliation, age or where they go for treatment.

Scarcely a person in this country has been untouched by this disease; either by a personal diagnosis or by knowing and loving someone who has had cancer. This disease must be combated psychologically and emotionally, as well as physically.

At weSPARK, everyone can express their fears and concerns in a safe, understanding and loving environment. Thanks to the support of our community and awe-inspiring volunteers, Wendie's dream continues to be fulfilled every day.

Go to http://www.weSPARK.org for information about programs, events, community support, and ways you can donate to this worthy cause.

weSPARK Sherman Oaks
13520 Ventura Boulevard
Sherman Oaks, California
91423
TEL: 818-906-3022
FAX: 818-906-3021

Quick Order form

Share this powerful new book with a friend or family

Making the Breast of It
Overcoming Fear of Intimacy After Mastectomy
By Lea Yekutiel

Online orders: http://www.ilovemybreastcancer.com
Telephone orders: 818-501-5908
Postal orders: Who Am I Press, 4444 Hazeltine Ave. #229
Sherman Oaks, CA 91423, USA

Please ship _____ copies of this book.

Name _____

Street address _____

City _____ State _____ Zip _____

Country _____

Telephone _____

E-mail address _____

Sales tax: Please add 8.25% for shipping to California addresses.

We accept: Visa ____ Master Card ____ American Express ____

Card # _____ Expiration date _____ Security Code _____

Shipping by Air
U.S.: $5.00 for first book and $2.50 for each additional book.

International: $10.00 for first book and $5.00 for each additional book.

For information on workshops and ezine subscription:
Visit our Web Site at http://www.ilovemybreastcancer.com